MY FAMILY & OTHER ALLERGIES

Safe and scrumptious recipes for diverse diets

JULIE GRITTEN

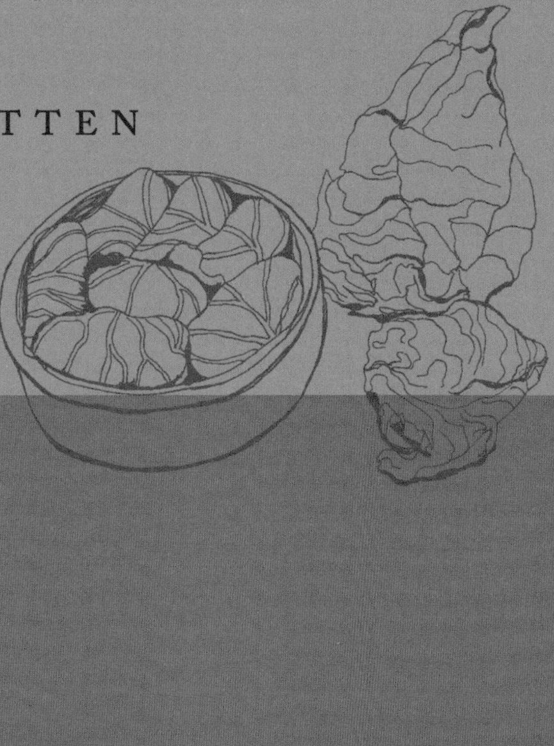

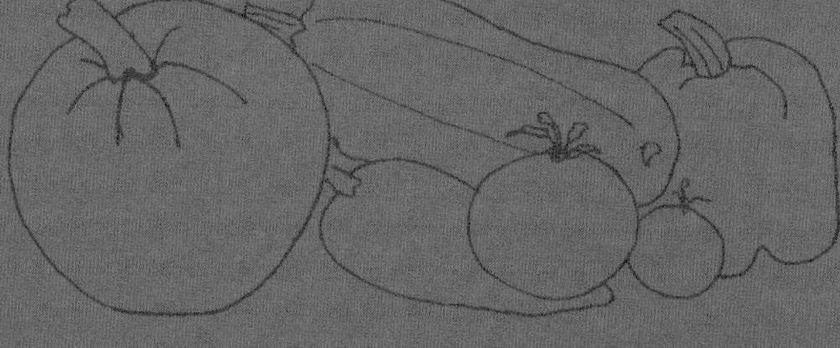

Hawthorn Press

Published by Hawthorn Press, Hawthorn House,
1 Lansdown Lane, Stroud, Gloucestershire, GL5 1BJ, UK
T: +44 (0)1453 757 040
E: info@hawthornpress.com
Website: www.hawthornpress.com

Illustrations by Julie Gritten
Design by Chris J Bailey
Printed by Henry Ling, The Dorset Press, UK
on environmentally friendly paper manufactured from renewable forest stock and other controlled sources.

FSC www.fsc.org MIX Paper | Supporting responsible forestry FSC™ C013985

British Library Cataloguing in Publication Data applied for
ISBN 978-1-912480-53-1

CONTENTS

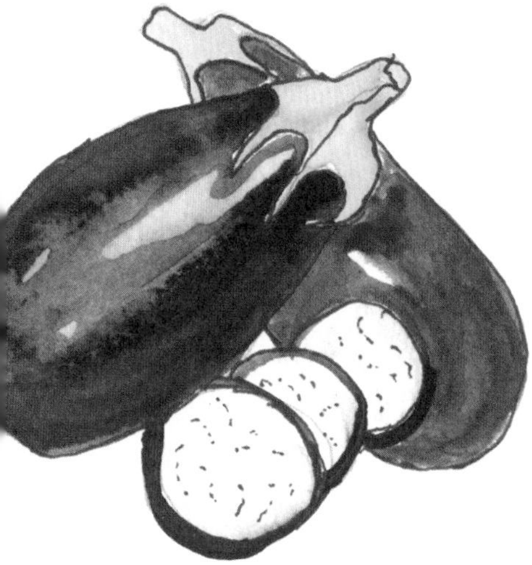

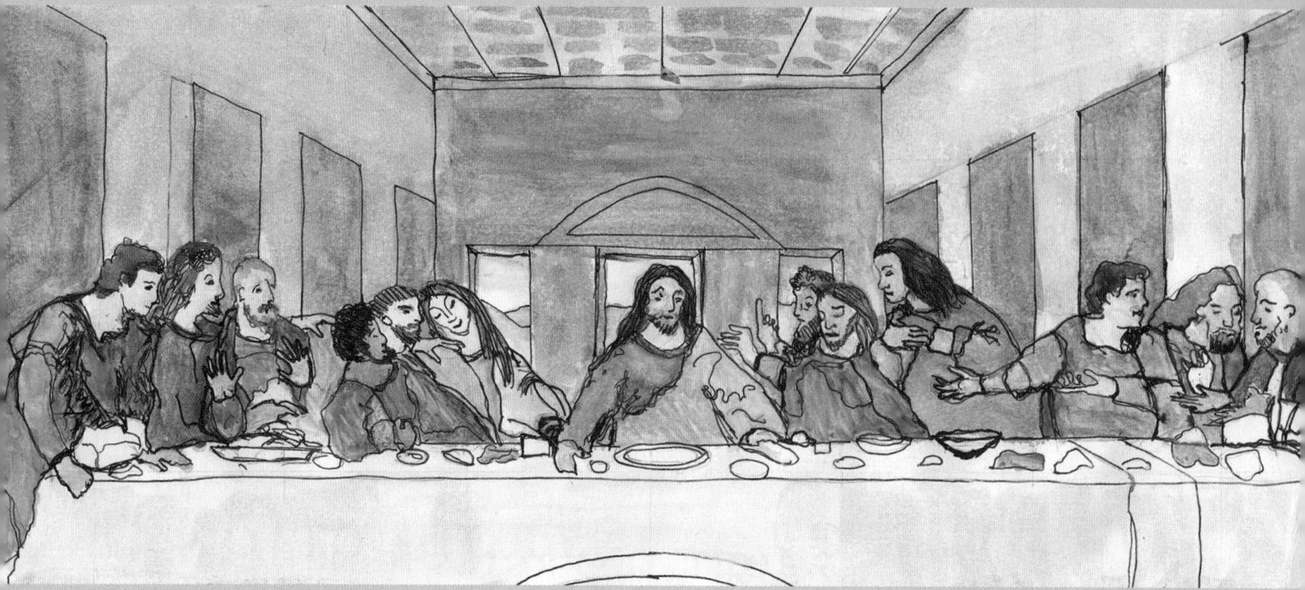

FOREWORD by Julie's only son, Wil

I don't have any issues with food. Was it a good move to ask the one person in the family with no food allergies to introduce a book about food allergies? Probably not.

My place at the table is one of omnivorous privilege from which I look down on all these fussy eaters with mild distaste.

I roll my eyes every time someone asks, 'Is there gluten in this?'

I growl when my hand gets slapped away from some delicious-looking salad because, 'That's for Gwen, not you.'

I barely even believe that food allergies exist at all.

But the nasty-looking sores Gwen gets from eating certain foods are real. The rashes and bad tempers my sister gets from even smelling oranges. The various stomach cramps, mouth ulcers and headaches that everyone apart from me suffers from. Those are real.

It's easy for me to imagine that everyone is making a big, unnecessary fuss because I don't understand the issues that affect them. That's the problem with privilege: people who are lucky enough to have it think that everyone who doesn't have it is just making a fuss.

What is at worst a mild irritation to me is a serious matter to them, the difference between happiness and misery. It is the imperative, therefore, that people like me should remain very aware of our luck and avoid indulging in lazy, harmful narratives. We have no moral option other than to behave compassionately and kindly, to embrace and accept that which we don't understand.

Julie, in her role as the Supreme Most Compassionate One, lays down an easy path to follow in this regard. Her ability to produce delicious meals that suit even the most allergic family members and visitors is astounding, and the results are delicious. She proves that cooking for people with food issues, including people like me whose only issue is other people's issues, doesn't have to be a limiting, compromising chore. She finds real joy in being adventurous with recipes, in meeting the challenge of omitting and replacing certain ingredients.

I have no doubt that this book will guide you down this same path, no matter how extreme the food issues that affect you, your friends or your family.

Thankfully, nobody is allergic to adventure and joy.

Bon appetit.

Wil Gritten, author of *Letting Go*

INTRODUCTION

Everybody eats differently but sometimes it's awkward cooking for those you care about.

Food is complicated. Everyone I know has some kind of complex relationship with food. I can't think of a single person, including myself and my family who doesn't think twice about eating one thing or another.

Many famous figures in history suffered from diet-related illness. Darwin had various gastrointestinal illnesses, picked up on his voyages around the world. Handel would grossly overeat and so suffered dyspepsia. During Queen Elizabeth I's final months, she refused to consume enough food or drink, which led to her becoming physically emaciated.

Celebrities such as Marilyn Monroe and Elvis had well recorded dietary issues and JFK, Eisenhower and Kurt Cobain are all said to have had IBS.

Whether we are vegetarian, vegan or meat eaters, whether we consider ourselves to have a healthy appetite or worry about our excessive intake, we give our minds, and our bodies, a lot to think about.

Once it was more simple – we ate what was gathered or hunted by the tribe. When times were hard there was less and we fasted and in times of plenty we feasted. Now we have a constant availability of food from everywhere in the world and we mix and match – an ingredient from China is mixed in the same dish as an ingredient from South

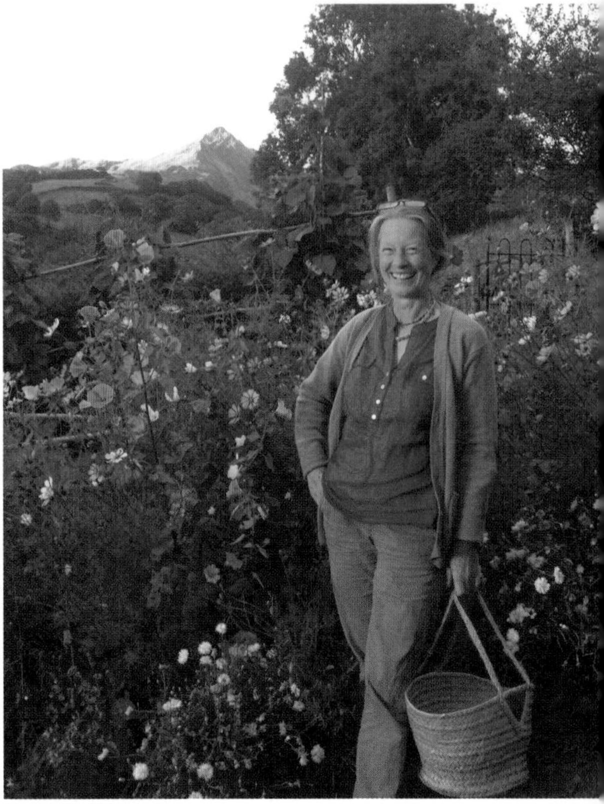

America. Now we eat manufactured foods and foods which contain totally artificial ingredients, prepared by machines.

Our current food industry was founded in the times of the British Empire and Industrial Revolution. The advent of great factories and mills brought people, who had worked the land, together to work machinery. Towns grew up around the mills and populations increased rapidly. To feed the growing number of working people, food became industrialised. Commercial canning, jamming and bread-making began in earnest. Sugar for instance moved from being a luxury to a necessity as our appetite for refined and adulterated foods grew.

This was reversed for a short time during World War II, when rationing led to a generation which grew up with little or no sugar. A generation which grew up on homegrown dug-for-victory vegetables, very little meat or dairy and free vitamin supplements. Rationing improved the health of British people, infant mortality fell and life expectancy rose.

But after the austere years of rationing, everyone needed a little extra. Extra sugar, extra chocolate, puddings and pies. Still the population was generally lean and meals were fairly simple – meat and two veg with a pudding and custard, sometimes washed down with milky tea.

Another sea change occurred in the 1980s when people began to put on weight in the era of fizzy drinks and hidden sugars in savoury foods. As a consequence many people, including children, suffer from type 2 diabetes, which was once a fairly rare condition of old age.

Now everything is more complicated. The number of people who have food intolerance or allergies has multiplied, with gluten allergy rising in particular. Vegetarianism and veganism has grown steadily and there are many people who choose to eat only local, sustainable, organic or raw food.

So what can we feed our loved ones, alongside ourselves? This book explains many of the reasons for our different food needs from ethics to the gut-brain axis. But more importantly it offers recipes alongside suggestions for putting it all together in a non-judging, harmonious way.

After all we all love to eat good food.

The old woman and her organic, spelt, sourdough bread

One day an old woman was sweeping her kitchen and found a five-pound note in a little crack in the floor.

'Aha' she said 'today I can buy myself a loaf of bread instead of making my own.'

So, she set off for the supermarket to buy her loaf.

When she got to the bread shelves, she could not find one single loaf which she could eat. There were wholemeal loaves and sliced bread, there were baguettes and cobs, but they all were inedible to her.

So, she called the assistant and said:

'Assistant, assistant, stock organic, spelt, sourdough bread or I shall not eat tonight!'

But would the assistant stock the bread?

No, he would not!

So, she called to the manager and she said:

'Manager, manager, help the assistant. Assistant won't stock organic, spelt, sourdough bread and I shall not eat tonight!

But would the manager help the assistant?

No, she would not!

So, she called the area managers and said:

'Area managers, area managers, educate the manager. Manager won't help assistant; assistant won't stock organic, spelt, sourdough bread and I shall not eat tonight!'

But would the area managers educate the manager?

No, they would not!

So, the old woman spoke to the supermarket owners and she said:

'Supermarket owners, supermarket owners, tell the area managers. Area managers won't educate the manager; manager won't help assistant; assistant won't stock organic, spelt, sourdough bread and I shall not eat tonight!'

But would the supermarket owners back the manager?

No, they would not!

So, the old woman called the newspapers and she said:

'Editors, editors, mount a campaign against the supermarket owners. Supermarket owners won't tell the area managers; area managers won't educate the manager; manager won't help the assistant; assistant won't stock organic, spelt, sourdough bread and I shall not eat tonight!'

But would the papers mount a campaign?

No, they would not!

So, she called all her friends and she said:

'Friends, friends, write to the editors! Editors won't mount a campaign against the supermarket owners; supermarket owners won't back the area managers; area managers won't educate the manager; manager won't help assistant; assistant won't stock organic, spelt, sourdough bread and I shall not eat tonight!'

And her friends said 'Yes, if we can tell all our friends to do it too?'

So, the old woman said:

'Yes, of course you can!'

As soon as everyone's friends had heard about it, the friends began to write to the editors, the editors began to mount a campaign against the supermarket owners, the supermarket owners began to tell the area managers, the area managers began to educate the manager, the manager began to help the assistant and the assistant began to stock the shelves with organic, spelt, sourdough bread

And the old woman bought a loaf and took it home to eat that night and it was delicious!

KEY TO SYMBOLS

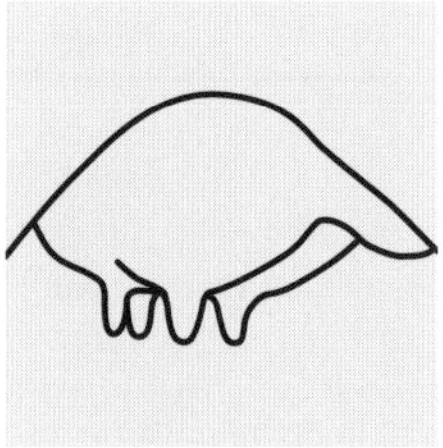
DAIRY

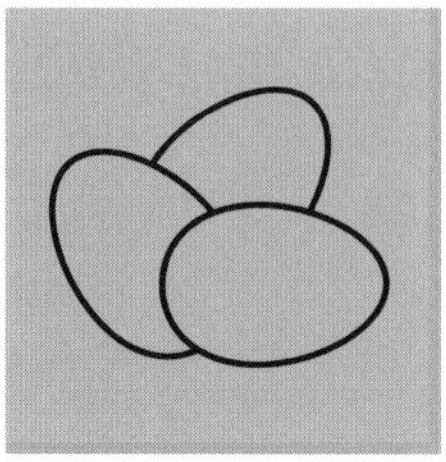
EGGS

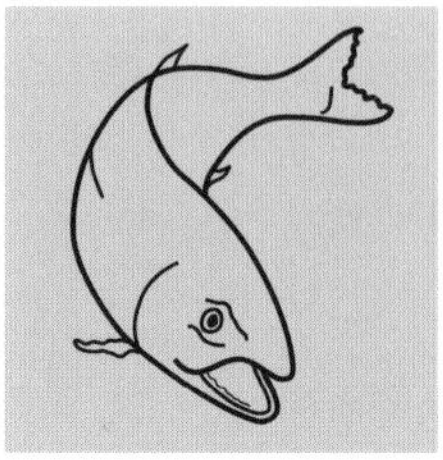
FISH

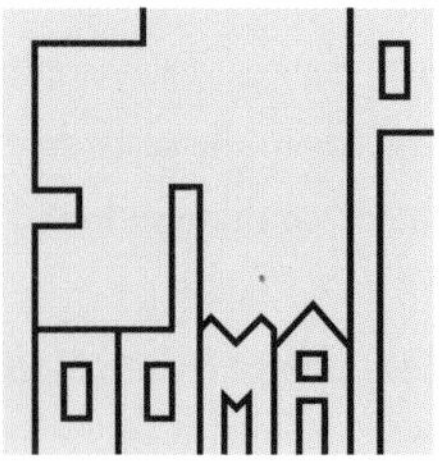
FODMAP

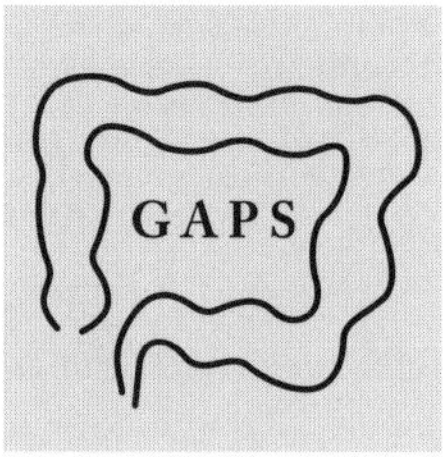

GAPS

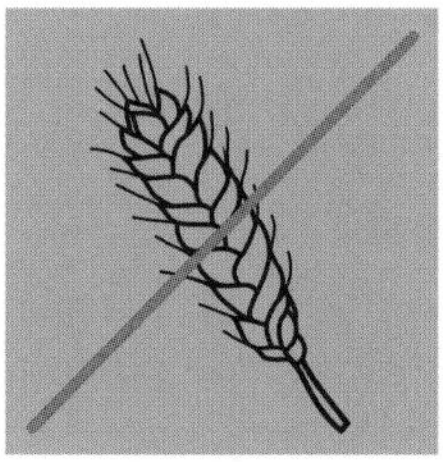
GLUTEN FREE

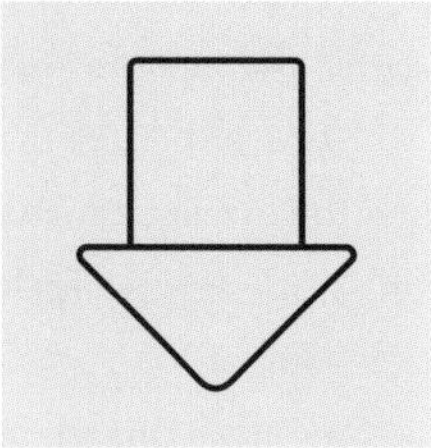
LOW SUGAR

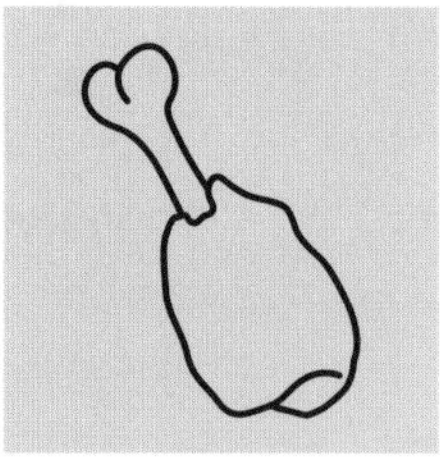
MEAT

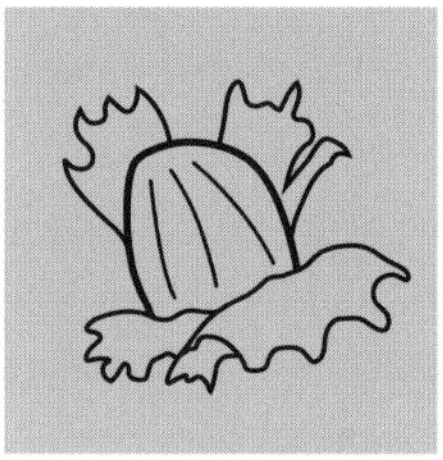
NUTS

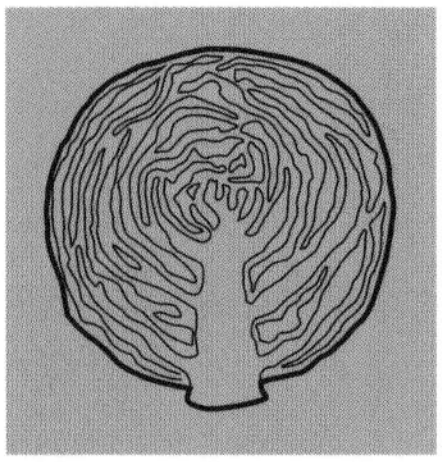
RAW

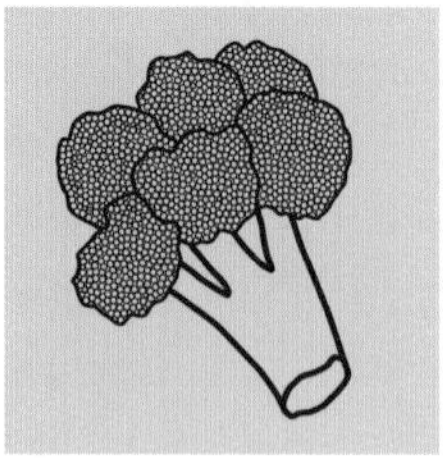
VEGAN

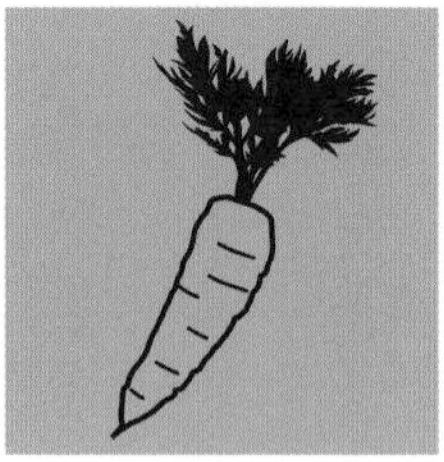
VEGETARIAN

THE PHYSICAL BODY

THE DIGESTIVE SYSTEM

We are basically doughnuts or polo mints.

That is, we have a hole running through us from top to bottom, and that long hole variously widens and narrows. There are pinch points (sphincters), a bag (the stomach), faster lanes and slower lanes. The function of this long hole is to process and break down what we put in our mouths into small elements that can be passed into our blood to be carted around the body for use and for the waste to be disposed of.

First we put the relatively large pieces of food into our mouths and chew. This begins to break it down and it is said that if we were to chew each mouthful 20 times we would have perfect digestion. Not many people adhere to this, though, and some of us hardly chew at all!

To help us break down food into component molecules, various chemicals are produced along the way – from the mouth, where cooked starch begins to be broken down, down through into the stomach, where acids and muscular churning break down the chewed food into a kind of soup. This 'soup' is then held by the stomach, which lets it out at intervals to be squeezed along the passageway of the small intestine, where various bits are further broken down.

As food components move along the small intestine (which can be up to 7 metres/23 feet long), they get broken down into smaller and smaller pieces until they eventually reach a sufficiently tiny size to allow each molecule to be absorbed through the wall of the small intestine.

Some digestive enzymes can only be found along the lower parts of the small intestine; for example, the enzyme responsible for digesting lactose (milk sugar). People with a milk intolerance are, in general, intolerant of lactose because they have a shortage or absence of this chemical.

Around 10 per cent of what we eat cannot be broken down to be absorbed by the small intestine so instead it passes into the large intestine to have the liquid sucked out of it, where it is stacked until it can be eliminated from the body as faecal matter.

The large intestine contains billions of bacteria known as the gut flora or gut biome. It has been estimated that we have more microbial cells than we have human cells in our bodies. These gut flora help with the breakdown process. In fact, around 30 per cent of your poo consists of these helpful bacteria. The bacteria in the gut also regulate the immune system, protect against bacteria that cause disease, and produce vitamins including vitamin B12, thiamine and riboflavin, and vitamin K.

Some of the bacteria are less helpful and when they overgrow or bloom it may result in a variety of problems, giving rise to symptoms such as bloating and excessive flatulence, symptoms of IBS or IBD and chronic constipation. There have been recent reports that unhelpful gut bacteria are complicit in Parkinson's disease, childhood leukaemia and Alzheimer's disease.

When the last 12 centimetres (4.5 inches) of the large intestines, known as the rectum, are packed with faeces, we open our bowels and poo.

We can positively affect our gut health by making sure we are eating a mixed diet with less meat (especially with less preserved meat) and plenty of fresh vegetables and a moderate amount of fruit.

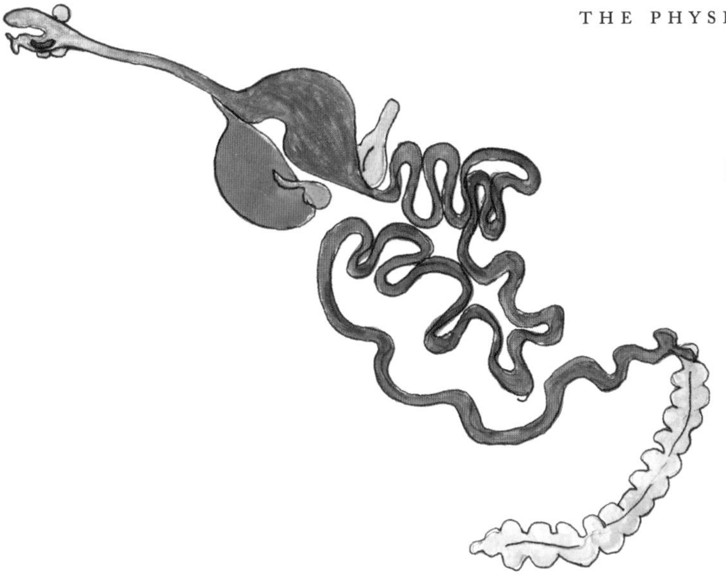

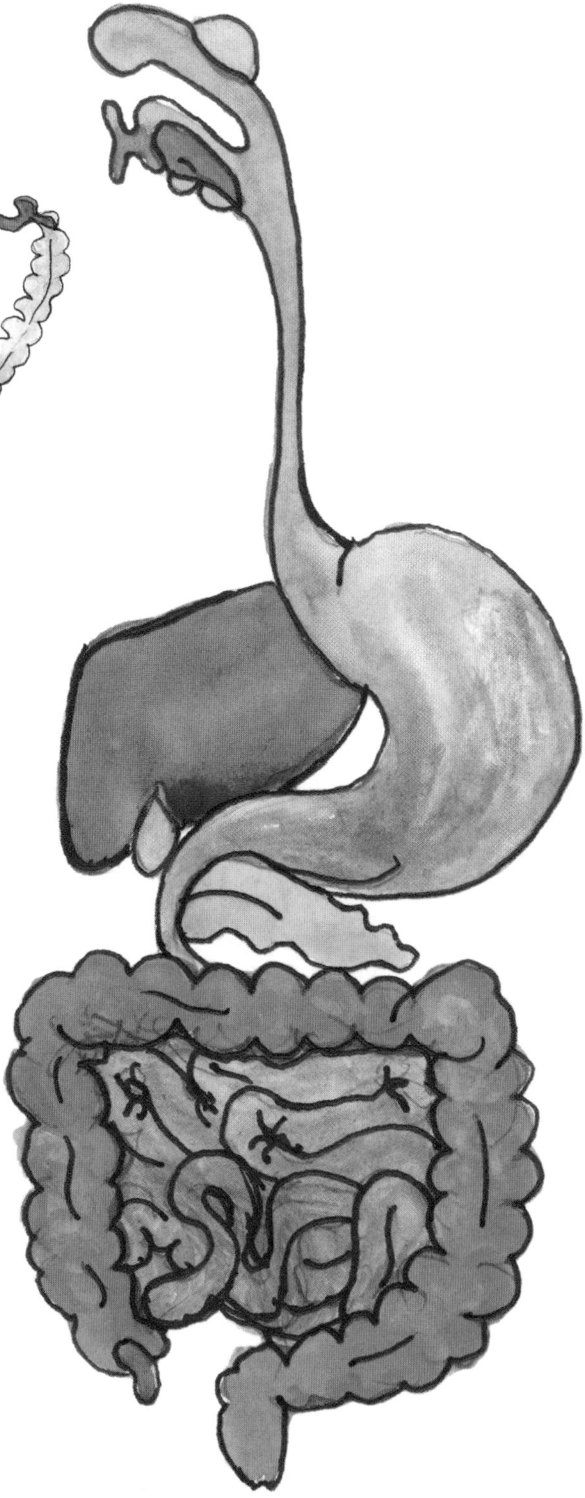

Laid out the digestive system comprises the lips; tongue and teeth; the mouth, salivary glands and gullet; oesophagus, stomach, pancreas and liver; the gall bladder and the small intestine, which can be up to seven metres (23ft) long; the colon (home to the gut biome) and then the appendix, rectum and anus.

It all fits neatly into the mid-body cavity that is formed in the first few days after conception. There is a constant rhythmic churning, causing stomach burps and belches, the borborygmi of the gut, the passing of wind, trumps and farts of the lower intestine and the raspberry-blowing of the anus. Flatulism was a professional entertainment act in Victorian times when people would fart out well-known tunes to enthusiastic applause.

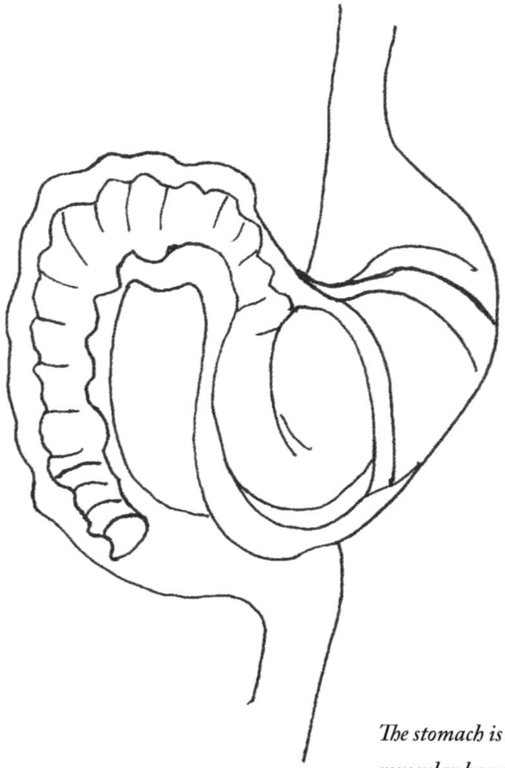

The stomach is a muscular bag which constantly churns and folds on itself to break down what you have swallowed. Gastric juices from the gall bladder and pancreas help to break down proteins, fats and fibre.

RECIPE

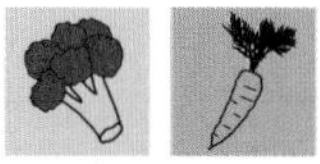

Sourdough starter

Wild yeast and lactobacillus in sourdough neutralise phytic acid (a cause of bloating and wind) as the bread proves. Sourdough bread acts as a prebiotic, which helps feed the good bacteria to help maintain a stable, healthy digestive system. It takes about a week for the sourdough starter to be ready.

- *225g (8oz) rye flour (check it is gluten free), plus 600g (1lb 5oz), divided*
- *250ml (8fl oz) cold water*

Mix the 225g (8oz) rye flour with the water in a mixing bowl until soupy, cover with a piece of cheesecloth or a clean tea towel and leave it to stand for a day.

Next day, add 100g (3½oz) of rye flour and enough water to return the mix to its soupy state. Repeat daily until all the flour is used up. Then split the mix into three and use two-thirds of it to start your bread and keep one-third as your starter to begin again.

You can keep the one-third of the mix in a sealed jar in the fridge until you are ready for more bread, then simply add 600g (1lb 5oz) of rye flour and enough water to make the mix soupy, then divide the mix as above and put the portion for keeping in a jar. I have successfully revitalised a starter after months of neglect.

You can make the sourdough bread with rye, spelt or wheat added to this rye starter (see page 82 for Homemade Rye Bread).

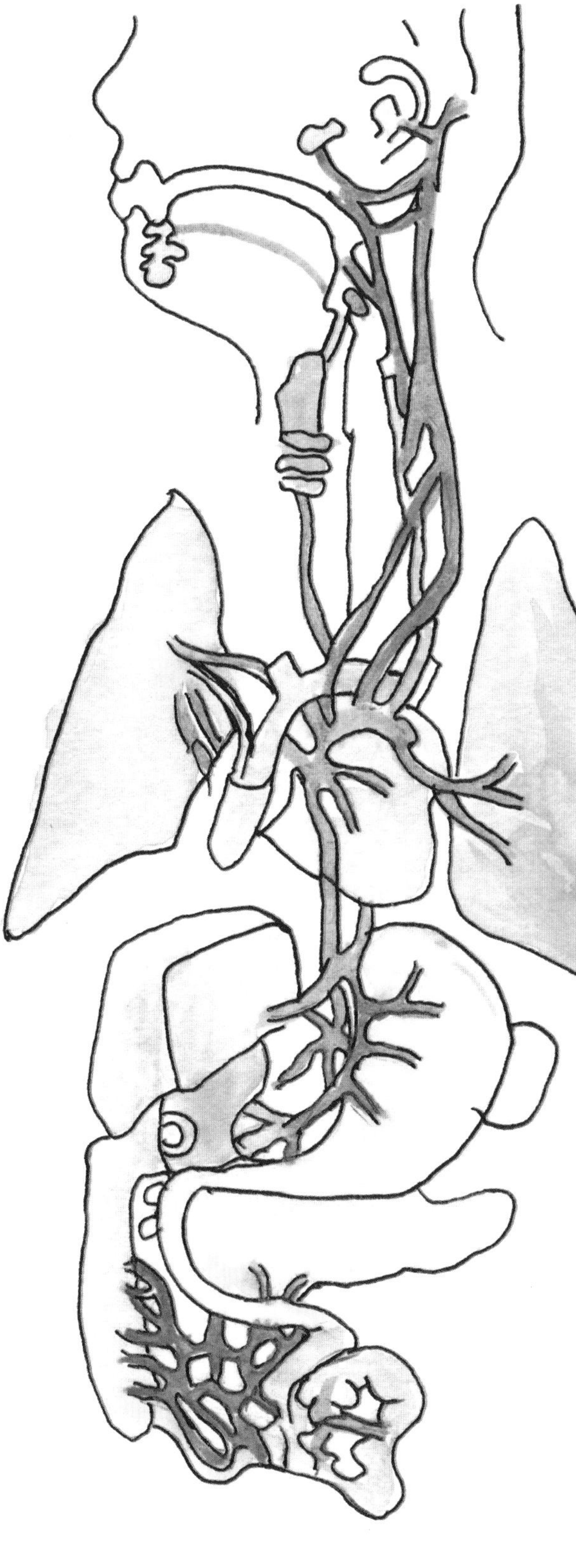

Diagram showing the complex pathways of the vagus as it wanders through the various organs of the body.

THE VAGUS NERVE

'The word vagus comes from the same stem as vagabond, meaning wandering… The vagus is the most complex nerve descending from the brain. It runs all the way through our bodies from tip to toe and touches everything. In a way it's the nerve that holds us together, connects us up, links all our individual parts, brains, lungs, hearts. The vagus nerve connects us to ourselves and if it gets broken it's the end of us. If we were puppets the vagus would be our strings.'

Tracks: The Nervus Vagus, Matthew Broughton, BBC Radio 4, 2016

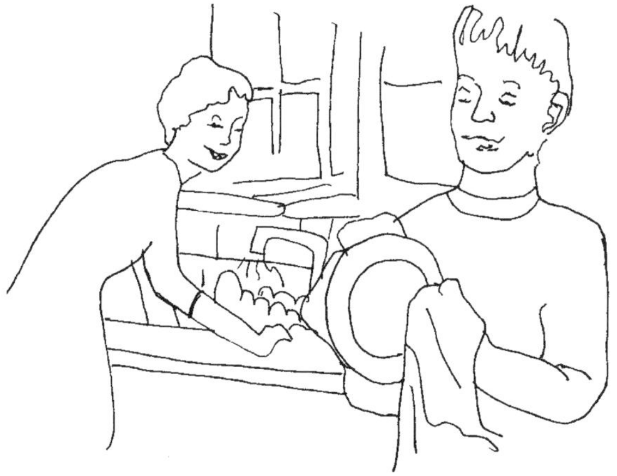

Mum, can drying up really help my vagus to switch on?

When I first learned about all the functions of the vagus nerve, I fairly fell in love with it (falling in love is a function of the vagus nerve) and wanted to write a book to tell the world all about it. The Latin word vagus means 'wandering' (the words vagrant and vague come from the same root).

The vagus nerve starts in the brain and extends all the way down to the colon, deep in the gut via the neck, chest and abdomen, so it is involved with the activities and health of the mouth, throat, chest, lungs, heart, stomach and intestine. In women it extends to the uterus and vagina too.

Among other things the vagus sends information about the state of the body's organs to the central nervous system. In the mouth it is involved with muscle movements for speech and for the secretion of saliva. It also has some control of our mouth muscles in chewing, swallowing and singing: the vagus helps us sing for our supper and then helps us eat and digest that supper.

The vagus stimulates the stomach to secrete acid and a protein called intrinsic factor. Intrinsic factor is needed to absorb vitamin B12 from food (which helps to maintain the nervous system and blood iron levels). It also plays a role in feeling satisfied after eating.

Vagus nerve fibres in the back of the throat are responsible for the gag reflex and vagus stimulation in the gut, has been shown to be a cause of vomiting.

A healthy or stimulated vagus function is known to reduce inflammatory illness and to switch the body from high anxiety 'flight or fight' to a 'rest and relax' state. Certain anti-inflammatory foods can help bring about this resting state by stimulating the vagus.

The vagus nerve is responsible for such varied tasks as heart rate and gastrointestinal peristalsis (the movement of food through the length of the gut).

The vagus has different branches which can effectively raise or lower blood pressure and lower or raise heart rate. In healthy people the activity of these two branches is balanced. It is this function that gives some of the emotional and physical effects that arise from sudden stress, such as feeling that your heart has stopped.

The old method of bringing someone round after a shock – by throwing cold water on them – stimulates the vagus nerve, which then causes the liver to produce insulin, which stops sugar production and slows the body and mind.

Other ways to stimulate the vagus are holding the breath

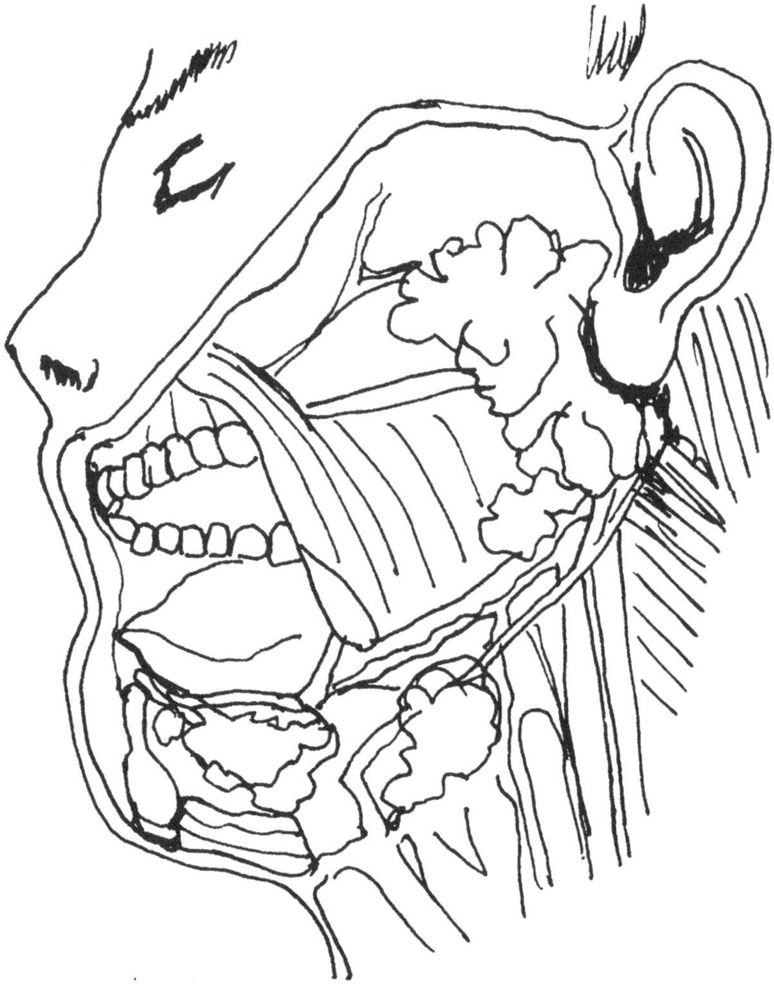

A section through the head shows the lines of the vagus nerve running up the back of the throat and the jaw line, past the fluffy-ooking salivary glands toward the ear.

for a few seconds, dipping the face in cold water and coughing or tensing the stomach muscles as if to bear down to have a bowel movement.

It has been said that in some cases, Parkinson's disease begins in the gastrointestinal tract and spreads via the vagus to the brain. Parkinson's disease is less prevalent amongst people who have had their appendix removed. It seems that it is a rogue gut bacterium that is partly responsible for the condition. The bacterium or its accompanying protein travels along the vagus nerve from the appendix to the brain, where it interferes with normal brain processes. It is better for you to have a healthy gut biome than have your appendix out! Rather than being vestigial, it appears that a healthy appendix acts as a reservoir for gut bacteria which can reseed the gut after a bout of severe diarrhoea.

Perhaps the vagus nerve is at the centre of much food intolerance and the symptoms of irritable bowel syndrome and other symptomatic gut disorders. It has some fibres in the inner tickly part of the outer ear and is involved with sweating. Some people get tickly ears when they eat something they are intolerant to, and many people sweat after eating hot curries or pickles. The vagus is involved in the breath, hence the symptom of wheeziness; the heart, hence the symptom of racing pulse; the brain, hence headaches.

The vagus may also play a major role in inflammation and various chronic diseases, if it is not working in a properly balanced way. So perhaps the root of allergic reactions to quite mild elements are also commanded by the vagus nerve.

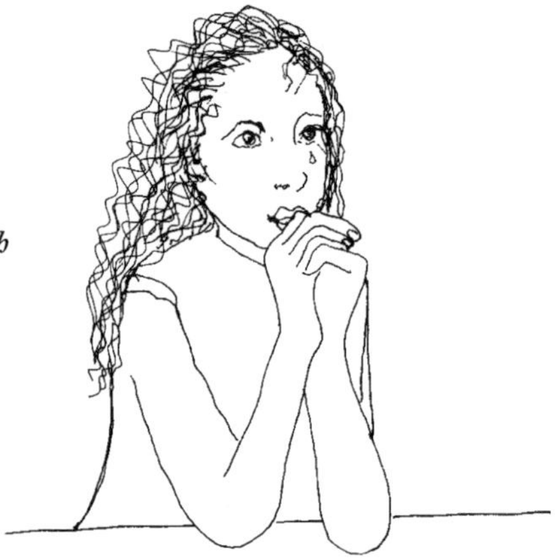

My vagus has gone for a wander and oh how I miss it

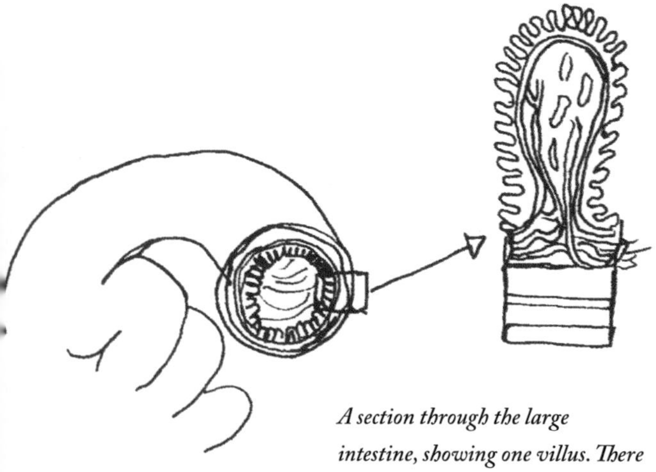

A section through the large intestine, showing one villus. There are neuropods on many of the villi, which connect to the vagus nerve. These neuropods trigger the vagus in response to various stimuli from the foods we eat and the gut biome.

And this fits in with the idea that much of our mistaken immune responses (such as allergic reactions and intolerance symptoms) follow illness, antibiotics or, according to some, vaccination, which all affect the vagus nerve.

As part of the parasympathetic system, the vagus allows the body to 'rest and digest', to enable your body to better respond to and recover from stress.

Vagus Nerve Stimulation – where a 'pulse generator' sends pulses of electrical energy to the brain – is used to help enhance the function of the vagus nerve, and one side-effect of such stimulation is laughter. In rare cases, too much laughter can cause fainting from overstimulation of the nerve.

The vagus affects our gut biome and vice versa. One of the probiotic bacteria of the gut, *Lactobacillus rhamnosus*, helps to achieve perfect levels of receptors of the calming chemical GABA (Gamma aminobutyric acid), which is mediated by the vagus nerve. Fermented foods, such as kimchi and sauerkraut (see pages 100 and 101) and beet kvass are probiotics that you can make at home.

Prebiotics, food for the colon cells, are found in fibrous vegetables. It is said that six or more servings of a variety of vegetables each day help to optimise the health of your gut biome, colon and vagus nerve.

Various microbiotics, such as the omega-3 fatty acids eicosapentaenoic acid (EPA) found in chia seeds, Brussels sprouts, hemp seeds, walnuts and flaxseeds, and docosahexaenoic acid (DHA), are found in seafood and are known to reduce inflammation in the body, and stimulate the vagus nerve to increase heart rate variability and lower the heart rate.

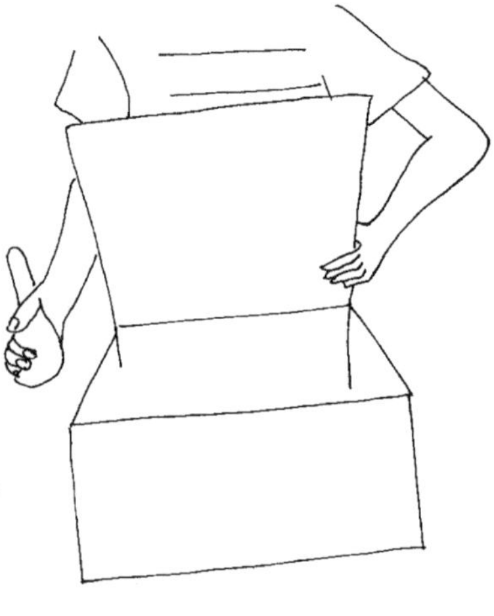

The vagus is the whole box of tricks that connects our bodies, heads, hearts and hands.

ABOUT ALLERGIES

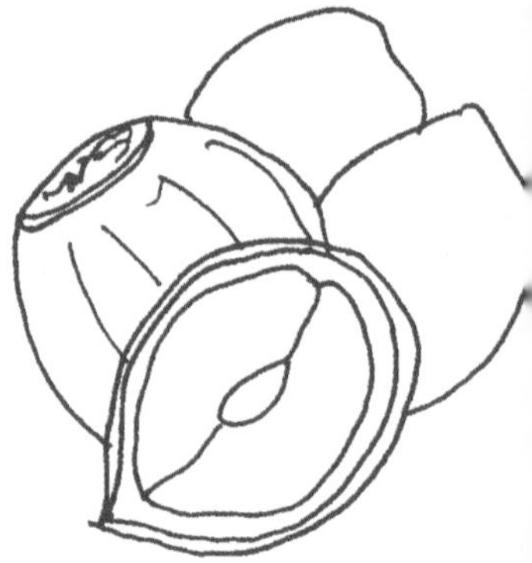

ALLERGIES

An allergy is caused by the immune system fighting substances in the environment that could be seen, by the majority of people, to be harmless.

The symptoms of mild to moderate food allergy include itching, burning and swelling around the mouth, swelling of the face or eyes, runny nose, skin rash and eczema, hives, diarrhoea, abdominal cramps, breathing difficulties, including wheezing and asthma, vomiting and nausea.

Some of the most common foods causing allergy in children are milk, eggs, peanuts, tree nuts, sesame seeds, fish and shellfish.

Jean

Jean has asthma, which she doesn't think is related to her diet. However, since she was around 13 or 14 years old, she has had an allergy to mushrooms. It may be genetic, as her brother has similar but milder symptoms, but her parents do not suffer at all.

It isn't so severe that she has to carry an EpiPen with her, and she has never been tested. However, she doesn't need a test to know that she should avoid mushrooms if she wants to avoid severe symptoms. She says, 'I suffer very painful bloating, so much so that I look pregnant, and have diarrhoea within about 20 minutes of eating even small amounts, as in a Bolognese sauce. Eating out isn't a problem. It's not so bad that pans or kitchen utensils have to be mushroom-free, and my symptoms have always been gastric, it's never set my asthma off. As far as I know it hasn't escalated, but I haven't eaten them in a long time.'

When eating out Jean has learned to avoid foods such as chicken pies, steaks, lasagne and anything that might contain mushrooms, and vegetarian food with Quorn in it also brings on symptoms. Jean has never had problems dining with friends and family and her favourite food is mac and cheese with bacon, for that umami flavour she misses by not eating fungi.

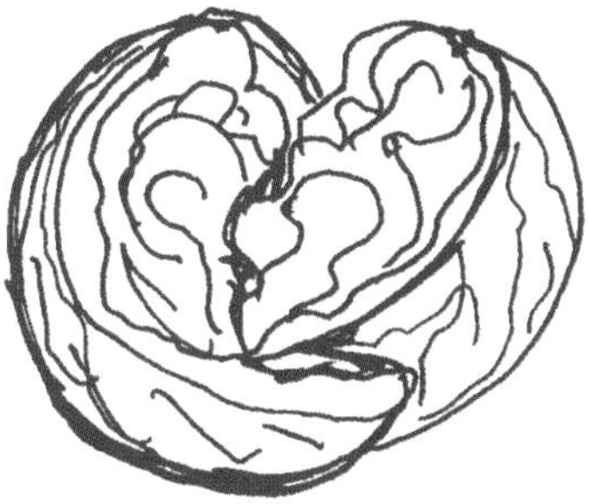

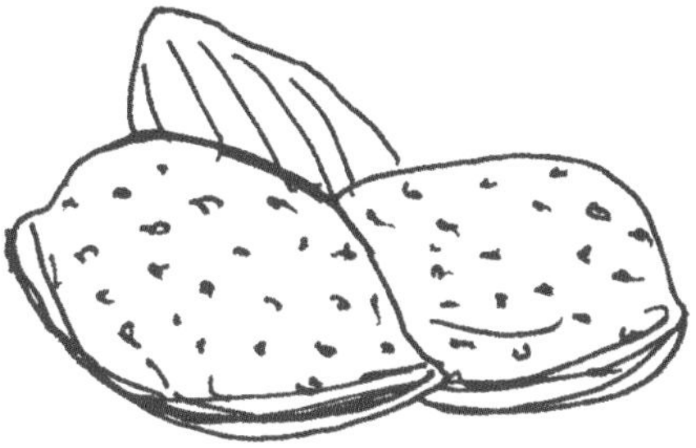

Not everyone has a problem with Almonds, as they are not nuts but kernels. Peanuts are not tree nuts but grow in the ground and are the most common allergen.

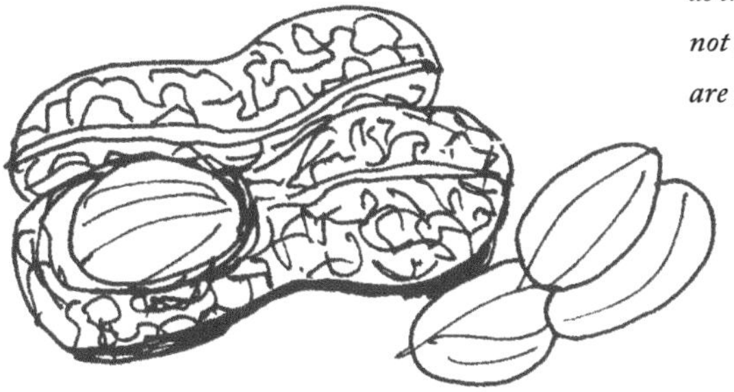

Jarret

Jarret is a keen and successful sea fisherman. He will eat pollock if he catches it, because he doesn't waste the bounty of the sea, but he has noticed that this doesn't always agree with him. He says, 'After eating a pollock ceviche [raw fish in lemon juice] my lips grew itchy, then my neck and chest. It lasted the whole evening and all night and then disappeared. It hasn't returned, though I did once eat a bad mussel which had similar results.'

This reaction has all the hallmark signs of allergy, which can appear at any age. Someone may never have had an allergic response to seafood before and suddenly have a severe reaction.

Jarret was lucky in that the symptoms did not persist and turn into a full-blown allergy.

Food allergy is nothing new, Hippocrates (460 BCE) noticed that cow's milk was associated with gastric upset and a rash. Galen (216 BCE) noted intolerance to goat's milk and Lucretius (95–55 BCE) said, 'What may be food to one may be fierce poison to others.'

In 1923, Coca and Cooke coined the term 'atopy' to describe hypersensitivity in humans. They considered atopy to be:

- hereditary and limited to a small group of people
- an abnormal response occurring in certain individuals (atopic)
- associated with an immediate type of skin reaction (wheal and flare)

Following Coca and Cooke's work, other studies reported the classic atopic diseases and the close association of asthma, hay fever, perennial rhinitis, atopic dermatitis and food allergies. The risk of a child developing an allergy is 40–60 per cent if both parents are atopic and 5–10 per cent if neither has any known allergies.

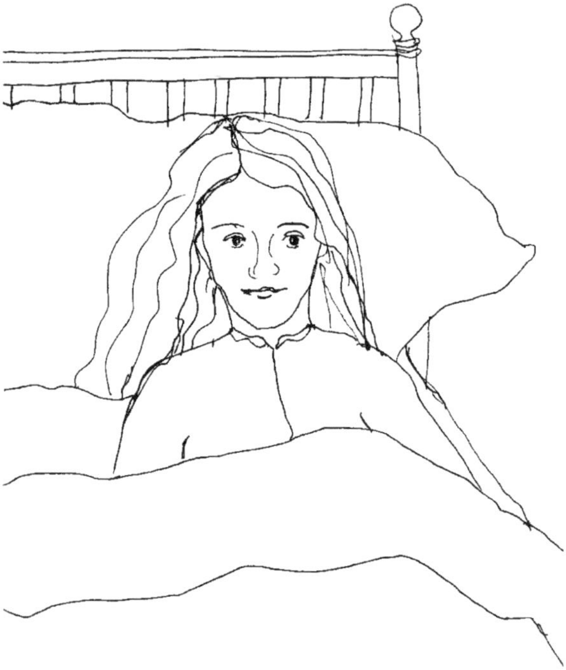

Louise

Louise is a meat eater because she is allergic to most fruit and some veg. It all started with a dairy allergy when she was eight years old and, it became progressively worse over the years.

She discovered her allergy to dairy because she frequently felt ill and as though she would faint after eating it. Testing then revealed that she had other allergies, and that the fruits and veg she didn't like were in fact allergy triggers. Her allergies to fruit and vegetables are related to pollen, though her response to dairy doesn't seem to be.

Louise's mum and sister are coeliac, her brother is allergic to milk and her dad is allergic to shellfish, so Louise doesn't often eat the same as the rest of her family do as it's too hard to accommodate all the family allergies.

Louise admits, 'I am able to eat out but am very restricted, I always choose the same dish in restaurants. I get lots of teasing and comments as it's a real pain in the ass for people.

Severe allergic reactions to foods can be life-threatening. Anaphylaxis is a severe allergic reaction that needs urgent medical attention. Foods such as peanuts, tree nuts, seafood, wheat, milk and eggs, as well as insect bites and stings and some medicines are the most common allergens that cause anaphylaxis. Within minutes of exposure to the allergen, the person can have potentially life-threatening symptoms, which may include difficult or noisy breathing, swelling of the tongue, swelling or tightness in the throat, difficulty talking, hoarse voice, wheezing, coughing, persistent dizziness or collapse or becoming pale and floppy (in young children).

Several factors can influence the severity of anaphylaxis, including how much exercise the individual takes, heat, alcohol, the amount of food eaten, and how food is prepared and consumed.

The frequency of allergic reactions to food has increased significantly over the past 30 years, particularly in industrialised societies. It is thought that these allergies and increased sensitivities are probably environmental and related to Western lifestyles. Fatal reactions are rare but they are also impossible to predict. To prevent severe injury or death, a person with anaphylaxis requires an injection of adrenaline (epinephrine), which can be given via an EpiPen.

Around 7 per cent of children in the UK suffer from food allergies and there was a five-fold increase in peanut allergies in particular in the UK between 1995 and 2016. The increase in allergies is not simply the effect of society becoming more aware of them and better at diagnosing them, but it may also be a result of factors such as increased pollution, dietary changes and less exposure to microbes, which change how our immune systems respond.

Pete

Pete has an allergy to raw mango, although he doesn't react to cooked mango, as in mango chutney. He thinks that perhaps the cooking denatures the chemical that he reacts to: 'I don't really take precautions because I can taste it before I consume too much. However, once I realised what the issue was, I stopped eating it, even though I like it dried!'

Like many people who have infrequent, non-threatening symptoms to certain foods, Pete hasn't had this allergy officially diagnosed. He has made some impromptu research, though, and looked up other members of the mango family such as cashew nuts, but he says, 'I haven't noticed any reaction to eating a handful of cashews, yet raw mango gives me a reaction with a 1cm or less square.'

This book includes some recipes using nuts or nut products. If you are cooking for someone with a nut allergy you must:

- ensure there are no nuts, peanuts or nut oils around when you prepare, cook and serve the food.
- read all labels very carefully.
- keep separate machines, implements, chopping boards, bowls and pans for use.
- warn your guests that there may be possible contamination if they eat with you.
- accept with grace that they may choose to not eat what you have prepared, if they are concerned.

There are seed and sesame recipes in this book, too, so if you are cooking for someone who has a sesame allergy it is best to follow the above advice and also keep all seeds in the cupboard along with nuts, just to be on the safe side.

And do be sure to check the ingredient lists very carefully on any pastes, masalas, ready-made sauces or food BEFORE you add them to dishes or serve them.

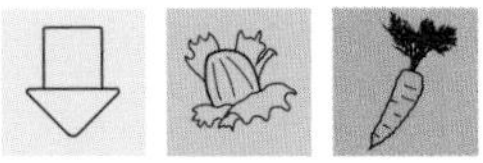

Anglesey no eggs

moderate oven & grill

serves 4

This is a good alternative to fish pie or Anglesey eggs for those who suffer from egg allergy.

- *450g (1lb) chopped leeks*
- *225g (8oz) fennel bulb*
- *475ml (16fl oz) Herby white sauce (page xx)*
- *1 tbsp finely chopped rosemary*
- *salt and pepper*
- *450g (1lb) mashed potatoes or cauliflower*
- *25g (1oz) sesame seeds*

Heat the oven to 180°C/ fan160°C/350°F/Gas 4.

Chop the leeks and fennel into 5cm (2in) rings and steam them in a pan for around 10 minutes or until soft. Season and place them in the bottom of a deep baking dish.

Cover with the herby sauce, scatter over the rosemary, top with the mashed potatoes or cauliflower and bake for 30 minutes in the oven or until warmed through.

Scatter the sesame seeds over and put under a hot grill for 5 minutes until the top is golden brown.

Buckwheat eggless pancakes

stove top

No adult allergy to buckwheat has been recorded in the UK. This is an egg free take on a Breton crépe. Make a thin batter and use a hot pan.

- *110g (4oz) buckwheat flour*
- *½ tsp bicarbonate of soda (baking soda) (optional)*
- *pinch of salt*
- *oil, for frying*

Mix the buckwheat flour, bicarbonate of soda and salt in a large bowl and add enough water to create a smooth, thin batter.

Allow the batter to stand while heating enough oil to just cover the base of a hot frying pan.

Pour the batter while rolling the pan so it covers the whole base in a thin, even layer. Alternatively, use a fish slice to smear the batter. When the pancake is solid in the centre, flip it over and cook the other side.

These are best served straight from the pan with sweet or savoury toppings.

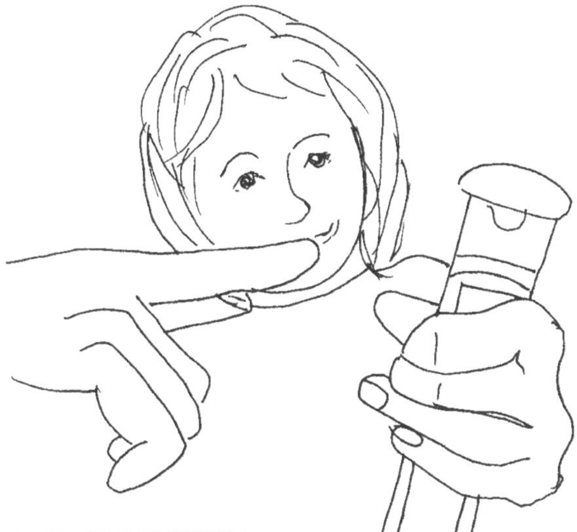

People have confidence in the EpiPen, although research suggests it may not be that successful if the allergy is severe. In less severe cases it is thought that there is a placebo effect.

Egg substitute 1

makes the equivalent of 1 large egg

This is good to use in vegan sweet recipes too.

- *2 tbsp water*
- *2 tsp baking powder*
- *1 tsp vegetable oil*

Mix everything together in a small bowl and use immediately.

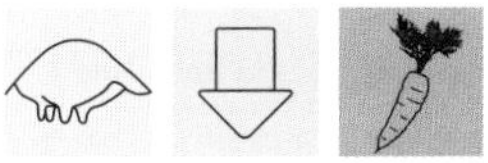

Herby white sauce

stove top

This is a really useful white sauce as you can use whichever ingredients present no challenges to your allergies. Use it in Anglesey No Eggs (see page 22) and over Steamed Vegetables (see page 64) or leave out the herbs and sweeten it to pour over fruit.

- *300ml (½ pint) milk or plant-based milk, plus 1 tbsp*
- *25g (1oz) plain, GF plain, corn or buckwheat flour*
- *1–2 tbsp chopped parsley*
- *salt and pepper*

In a cup, mix the 1 tablespoon of milk with the flour to make a paste.

Heat the rest of the milk in a pan until almost boiling. Remove from the heat and whisk in the flour mix, then return to the heat and stir continuously until boiling. Simmer for 2 minutes then add the parsley and seasoning to taste.

Lamb burgers

stove top

serves 4

This simple recipe makes tastier burgers than those bought at one of the biggest UK supermarkets, which listed the ingredients in theirs as: Lamb (84%), Water, Dried Potato, Rice Flour, Sugar, Mint, Flavouring, Parsley, Salt, Onion Powder, Paprika, Garlic Powder and Sodium Metabisulphite.

For this recipe, mince the lamb yourself, if you can, but if not pre-minced meat is fine.

- *450g (1lb) minced lamb*
- *1 onion, minced or finely chopped, plus extra fried, to serve (optional)*
- *1 egg, beaten*
- *1 tbsp finely chopped mint (optional)*
- *salt and pepper*
- *gluten-free buns, to serve*

In a large bowl, with your hands work all the ingredients together until the mix feels plump and holds together, then form the mix into burger shapes.

Fry or barbecue in the usual way on both sides until they are golden brown and the inside is well cooked.

Serve on a bun with fried onions, if you like.

Poached pears

moderate oven

serves 4 (+ 1 spare)

Pears are said to be one of the least allergenic foods. If sensitive to cinnamon, exchange it for star anise.

This works for poached quince, too, although they take longer to cook.

- *5 small pears, peeled, but stalk intact*
- *1 cinnamon stick*
- *1 tbsp sugar, agave, date or coconut syrup*
- *4 tbsp water*

Heat the oven to 180°C/ fan160°C/350°F/Gas 4.

Place the pears and cinnamon stick in an ovenproof dish. Add the sugar to the water and pour it over the pears.

Cover and place in the oven for 30 minutes, then remove the cover and cook for another half hour until the pears are tender when pierced with the tip of a sharp knife. Remove from the oven and allow to cool.

Transfer the pears to plates and, if there is any leftover syrup, boil it in a pan with the cinnamon stick until it is thick, then pour it over the pears.

Serve cold with the syrup and cream (soya or oat, if you prefer) or ice-cream.

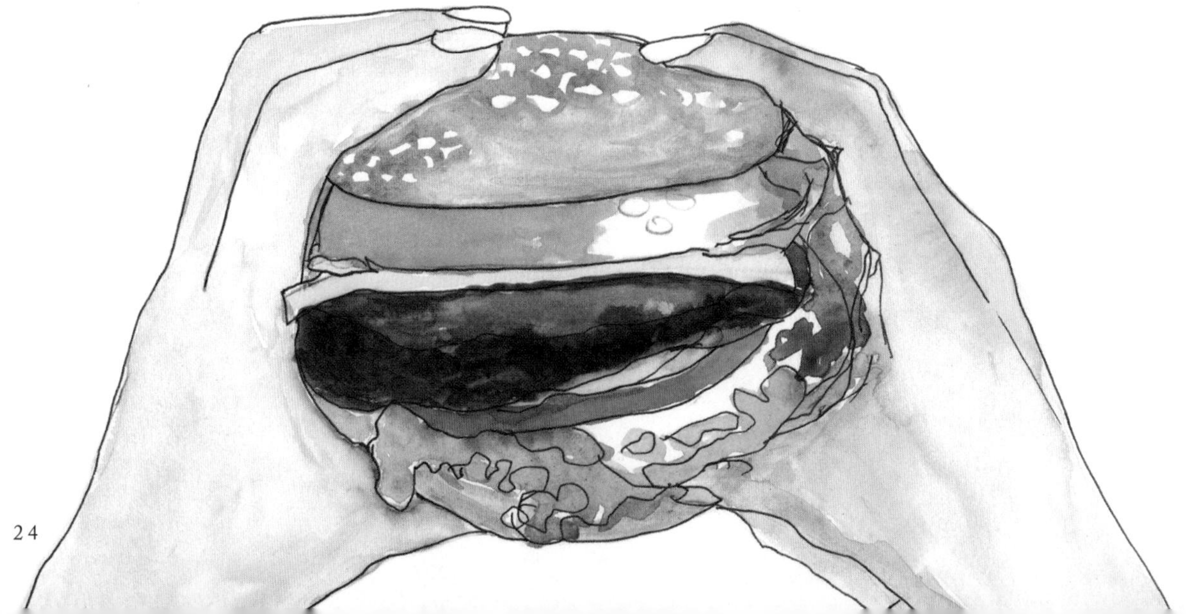

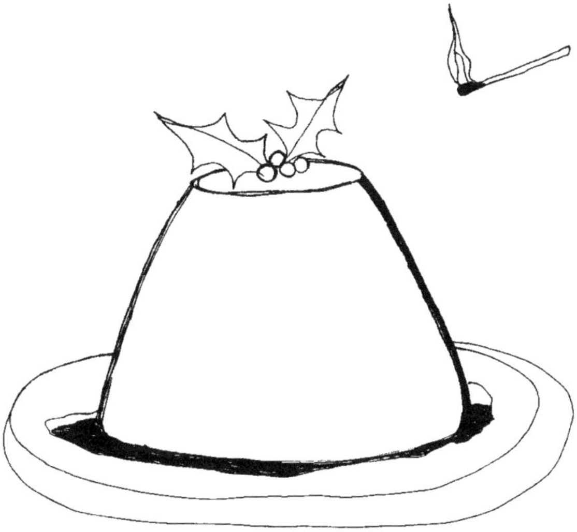

Christmas pudding

stove top

serves up to 8

This recipe puts you in complete control of what goes into the pudding, so substitute what you can't have for tasty alternatives such as ginger, cherries, prunes or dates. Make the pudding at least three weeks before Christmas. If you prefer, you can substitute some fruit or add crystallised ginger, cherries, prunes or dates.

- *225g (8oz) sultanas*
- *350g (12oz) raisins*
- *225g (8oz) gluten-free plain flour*
- *2 tsp mixed spice*
- *2 tsp ground cinnamon*
- *2 tsp grated nutmeg*
- *½ tsp salt*
- *120g (4½oz) soft brown sugar*
- *70g (3oz) ground almonds – or use more flour if not using almonds (optional)*
- *110g (4oz) currants*
- *3 eggs or the equivalent egg substitute (page 23)*
- *1 tbsp molasses*
- *About 4 tbsp water or ale*
- *1 tbsp brandy (optional)*

Mince the sultanas and raisins together or chop them until they are very small.

Sift the flour into a large bowl, then add the chopped dried fruit, spices and salt together, then add the sugar and almonds (or extra flour). Using your hands, rub everything together as for pastry.

Add the currants, eggs and molasses and beat the mix with a spoon. Add the liquid a spoonful at a time and beat to make a thick, dropping mix. Stir in the brandy, if using.

Pour the mixture into a greased pudding basin and cover with greaseproof paper and a pudding cloth or silver foil. Put the bowl in a steamer (use a pan with a foldout veg steamer at the base) and steam for 4 hours. The pudding will rise a little. Carefully remove from the steamer while still hot.

When cold, pour on a little more brandy and re-wrap the basin with fresh greaseproof paper and waxed cloth or cling film. The pudding will keep for at least 3 weeks.

On the day that you want to eat it, wrap the pudding as before and steam it for 3 hours. Serve with a sprig of holly on top and your cream of choice. It is traditional to pour warm brandy over the pudding and bring it flaming to the table – we always sing the Figgy Pudding song as we do so!

FOOD INTOLERANCE

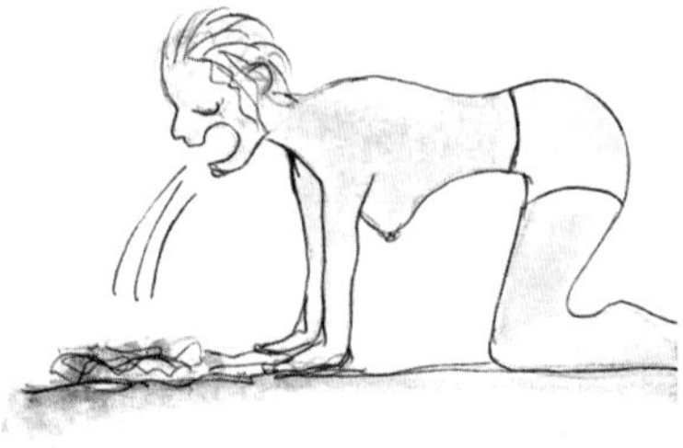

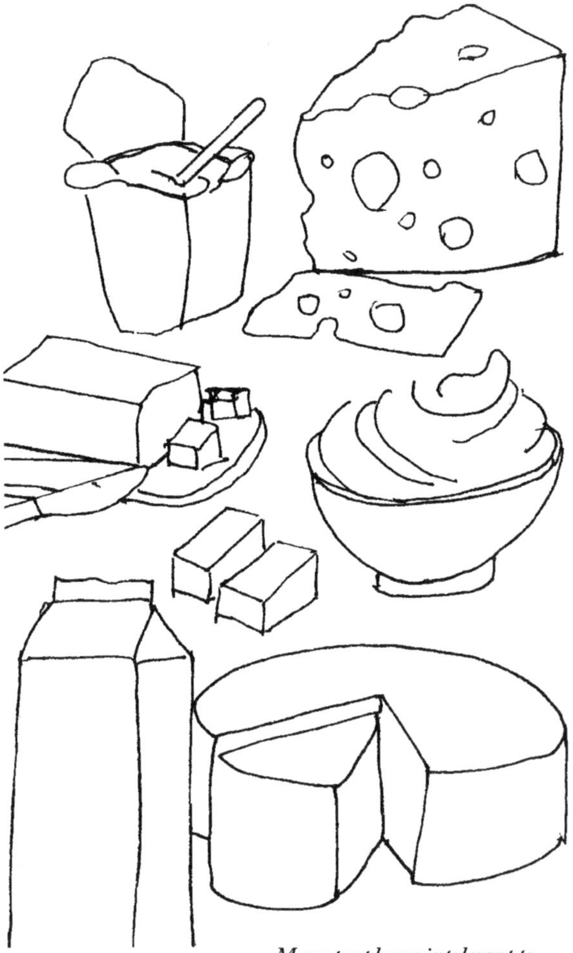

Many people are intolerant to milk and milk products. However, many of these can tolerate butter, yogurt and hard cheese.

Food intolerance symptoms can resemble those of food allergy. The difference is that food intolerance is not so severe as an allergy, doesn't involve the immune system, doesn't show up on allergy tests and doesn't lead to anaphylactic shock. Why we can be food intolerant is poorly understood by the medical world. By relations or friends it can be seen as being trendy. There has been a lot of chat online and in the press about people who eat gluten-free food but don't have coeliac disease.

Symptoms of food intolerance can include:

- **nervousness (mood swings, anxiety, paranoia, temper tantrums, acting up, crying and being over-emotional)**
- **tremor**
- **sweating**
- **palpitations**
- **rapid breathing**
- **headache, migraine**
- **diarrhoea**
- **constipation**
- **burning sensations on the skin**
- **tightness across the face and chest**
- **breathing problems**
- **asthma-like symptoms**
- **allergy-like reactions**
- **muscle and joint pain**

The habit of asking people what they can or would like to eat often brings up admittance of food intolerance which otherwise they would keep to themselves and suffer in silence.

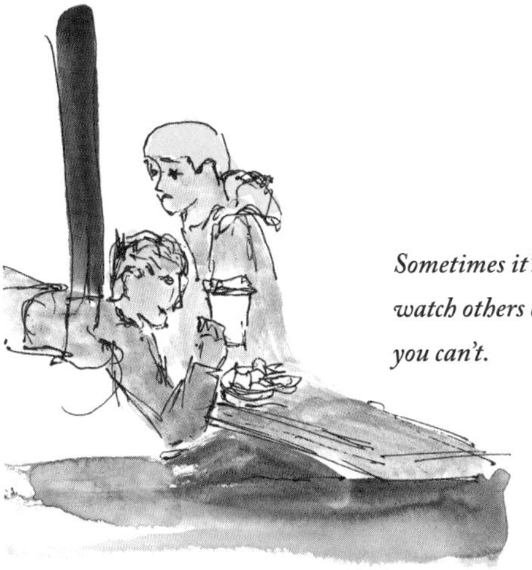

Sometimes it's hard to watch others eat what you can't.

The drink with that mystery ingredient! 'Oh no, I'm intolerant to mystery'

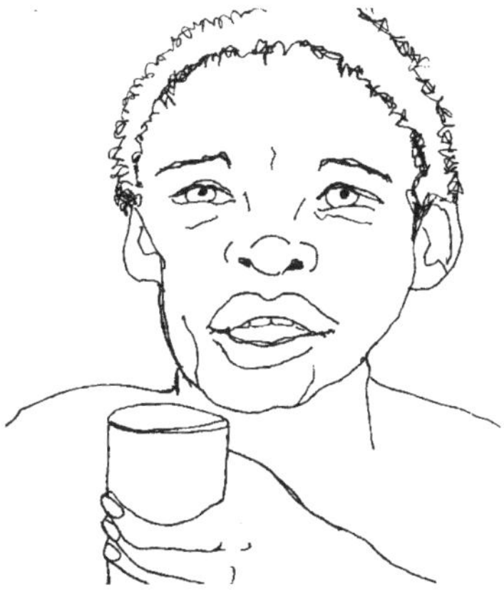

John

My partner John and I had been backpacking in Thailand and John went back to work the day after we arrived home, jet-lagged and tired. The next week was a bit of nightmare for him. A rash had broken out on his skin on either side of his waist and along the fronts of his thighs. The doctor suggested it was a sarcoptic mange, such as scabies.

Really, we should have treated the whole family, washed all the bed linen, cleaned the carpets and cushions, but no one else seemed affected or had symptoms except for John, so he had to bathe in a vile liquid to get rid of the parasites. Though he came out very, very clean it didn't seem to work and he still had the itches.

They began every evening around 6pm and went on until midnight but were gone the next morning. It carried on for another week but, after another visit to the doctor, John finally twigged that each evening he came home from work, he would have a chocolate bar and the itching would start a little while after. He stopped eating chocolate and he stopped itching almost immediately.

He gave up chocolate for almost two years and then had a little now and then. Now he can eat chocolate but occasionally I see him scratching his thighs and I give him the, 'Been eating chocolate?' look.

Marley

'Mam, the baby looks like a speckled hen's egg!'

Our baby Marley was born with spots. Little angry red spots covered her face and body. Just a newborn rash, we were told. Marley had colic and reflux and sometimes refused to breastfeed.

All through the pregnancy I had kept up with my vitamin and mineral intake by drinking a daily glass of orange juice with brewer's yeast and vitamin C with spirulina. I carried on with it after her birth until at three months old she utterly refused to accept my milk. I tasted it and it was sharp and acid and tasted of oranges.

Scroll back 20 or so years to me as a teenager. I was not spotty but I did have cold sores. All through the winter my lips would be lined with serious cold sores. I carried on having them throughout my student years and into motherhood. Sometimes huge and sometimes tiny, and accompanied by mouth ulcers, but almost always present. So it was like a little miracle that when I stopped eating oranges and drinking the juice for Marley's sake I stopped having cold sores. And my life without cold sores has been all smiles!

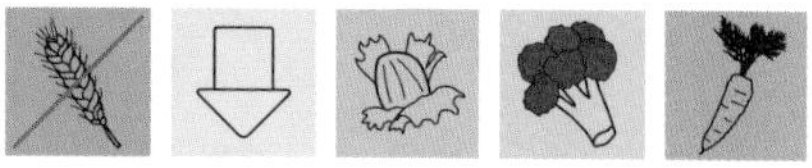

Crackers

moderate oven

makes 12

A plain, bought cracker may have many ingredients that cause you a mild upset or may set off a cascade of symptoms. Ingredients in one cracker include 'wheat flour, sunflower oil, sugar, glucose-fructose syrup, calcium phosphates, ammonium carbonates, sodium carbonates, potassium carbonates, salt, barley malt flour and dried yeast'. This recipe makes crackers that are tasty alternatives where you control the ingredients.

- *150g (5oz) gluten-free flour, plus extra for dusting*
- *110g (4oz) almond or buckwheat flour (buckwheat makes a slightly softer cracker)*
- *¼ tsp baking powder*
- *½ tsp garlic powder (optional)*
- *1 tsp finely chopped rosemary (optional)*
- *1 tbsp poppy seeds (optional)*
- *2 tbsp sunflower or rapeseed oil, plus extra for greasing*
- *5–8 tbsp cold water*
- *salt and pepper*

Oil or flour a baking sheet.

Mix all the dry ingredients thoroughly in a large mixing bowl then stir in the oil until the mix is crumbly. Add the water 1 tablespoon at a time, blending it in until the dough is mouldable. Roll out on a lightly floured surface to 3–5mm (¼in), between two sheets of baking paper.

Score the dough into small squares using the tip of a sharp knife. If the dough is very soft, keep it on the paper and transfer it on the tray to the freezer or fridge for 10 minutes until firm.

Heat the oven to 220°C/ fan200°C/425°F/Gas 7.

Using a spatula, transfer the crackers to the prepared baking sheet and bake for 15–20 minutes until golden.

Use within 3 days. If they soften, crisp them up by placing them in a warm oven for 5–10 minutes.

It's hard to discuss your food intolerance at the meal table

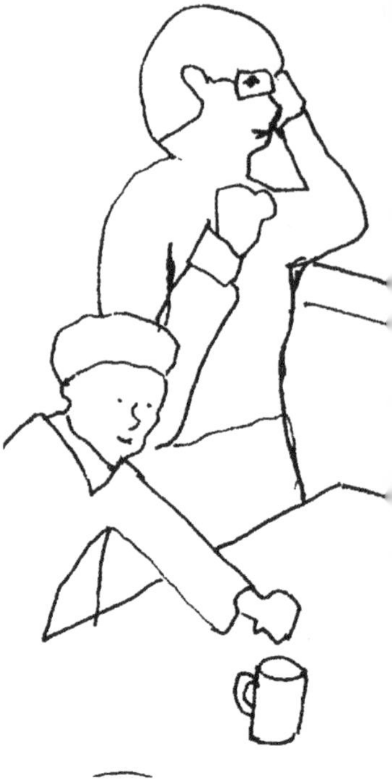

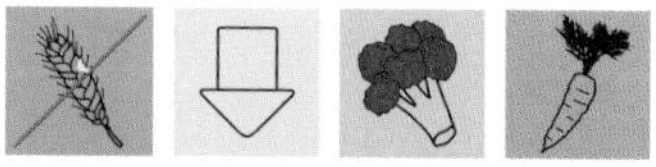

Chapatis / flatbreads

stove top

makes 6–8

We eat these as wraps, on picnics and when travelling. Wholemeal flour makes a less fluffy version. These are a good substitute for naan, which contain milk.

- *225g (8oz) white or wholemeal, spelt or gluten-free flour with ½ tsp xanthan gum, plus extra for dusting*
- *1 tsp salt*
- *100ml (3½ fl oz) lukewarm water*
- *1 tsp vegetable oil / coconut oil*

In a large mixing bowl, combine the flour and salt. Add the water a little at a time and, just as the mix begins to combine, add the oil and knead until firm and not sticky (add more flour or water as needed to make it into a smooth ball).

Divide the dough into even sized 3–4cm (1¼–1½in) balls and flatten them. On a floured board, roll them out into circles 1–2mm (⅛in) thick. The flatbreads are best if the dough is allowed to rest for 30 minutes before using.

In a hot, dry frying pan, cook the flatbreads on each side for up to a minute until puffy and browned.

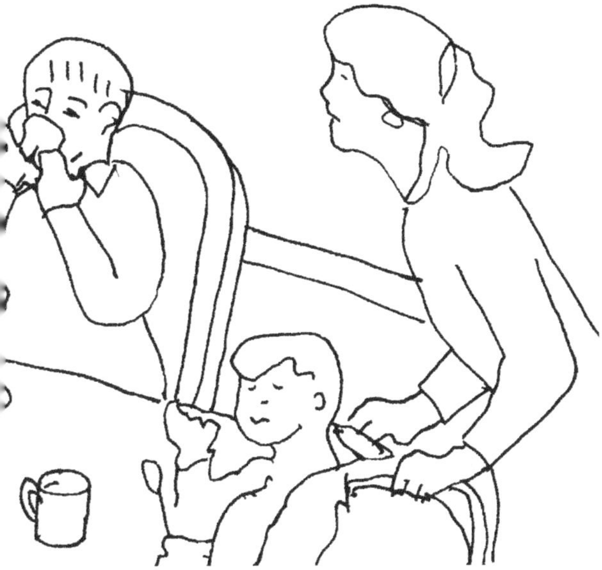

Hummus version 1

serves 4

Much hummus that you buy has ingredients you don't need, such as acidifier E330 (anhydrous citric acid) and preservative E202 (potassium sorbate) as well as sesame oil. If you are sensitive to sesame, leave it out of this recipe and add a drizzle of olive oil across the top.

- *1 tin cooked chickpeas drained, twice rinsed*
- *1 tbsp tahini (optional)*
- *1-2 garlic cloves*
- *Juice of 1 lemon / 1tbsp cider vinegar*
- *seasoning*
- *2 tbsp olive oil / water to soften mix*
- *1 tsp finely chopped parsley*

Blend all the ingredients till smooth, either by hand or with a blender. Add more vinegar or a little water if too thick. For a richer flavour, allow the hummus to mature overnight.

Make a smoother hummus by removing the chickpea skins.

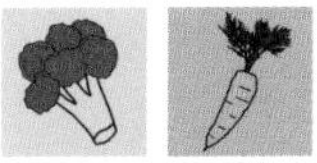

Scotch Megs

stove top

makes 2

My daughter Meg devised this recipe, which her children really enjoy. These are good for vegetarians and vegans as well as people who can't eat egg or are intolerant to the additives in sausage meat. Try fillings like feta cheese, marinated tofu, or roast tomato.

Filling

- *2 tbsp finely grated carrots*
- *2 tbsp finely grated courgette (zucchini)*
- *1 tsp dried mixed herbs*
- *1 tsp olive oil*
- *salt and pepper*

Coating

- *125g (4½oz) 'Sosmix', made up according to packet*
- *1 tsp tomato purée*
- *pinch of chopped basil*
- *pinch of grated nutmeg*
- *1 tsp garlic (optional)*
- *2 tbsp flour*
- *1 litre (1¾ pints) oil for deep-frying*
- *salt and black pepper*

Sauté all the filling ingredients together in a frying pan and add some seasoning. Leave to cool.

Once cool, with your hands form the mixture into 2cm (¾in) balls. Set to one side.

In a mixing bowl, combine the Sosmix, tomato purée, basil, nutmeg and garlic and season to taste.

Divide the mix evenly to make two Megs per person.

Flour your hands and place one portion of the filling mix in the middle of the coating mix. Close the coating up and seal tightly.

Roll each Scotch Meg in the flour and deep-fry in a wok or deep pan for about 15 minutes until golden brown all over and well cooked.

Serve hot or cold.

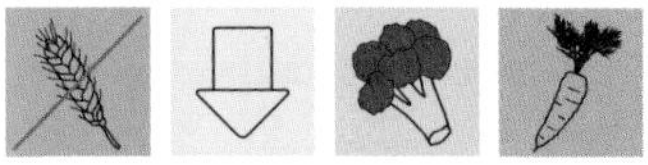

Nomato cooking sauce

stove top

serves 4

Symptoms of tomato intolerance sometimes show up as late as 72 hours after tomatoes have been eaten, so it takes a while to understand if you have a problem with them. If you think you may have, try this as an alternative sauce.

- *1 medium onion, finely chopped*
- *1 tbsp oil or cooking fat*
- *1 garlic clove (optional)*
- *1 medium beetroot, chopped*
- *2 medium carrots, chopped*
- *1 celery stalk, finely chopped*
- *1 courgette (zucchini), finely chopped*
- *1 tsp dried mixed herbs*
- *400ml (14fl oz) meat, berry or veg bouillon stock*
- *1 tbsp chopped basil*
- *salt and pepper*

Fry the onion in the fat or oil in a large saucepan, add the garlic and cook for about 5 minutes, until softened. Add the rest of veg and the mixed herbs and fry for further 5 minutes.

Add the stock and season, put a lid on and simmer for 20–30 minutes until all the vegetables are soft. Add a little more water if needed. Blend or mash the vegetables and stir in the basil, if using.

Serve with pasta or on dolmades (page 136).

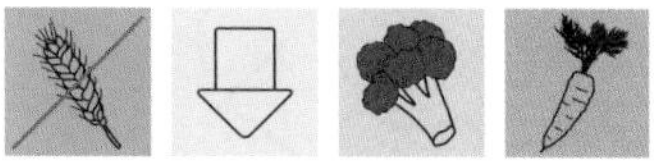

BBQ courgette

barbeque

per person

People with food intolerance to several things may find themselves missing out on the fun of a BBQ. Offer this to include them as courgette intolerance is rarely a problem. The courgettes can be cooked on a griddle instead of a barbecue.

- *1 courgette (zucchini)*
- *1 tbsp olive oil*

Olive oil dressing (optional)

- *1 tbsp lemon juice or cider vinegar*
- *1 tbsp olive oil*
- *salt and pepper*

Slice the courgette in quarters lengthways. Brush the quarters with oil and barbecue them for 5 minutes on each side or until brown and stripy. Place in a dish and pour over the olive oil dressing, if using.

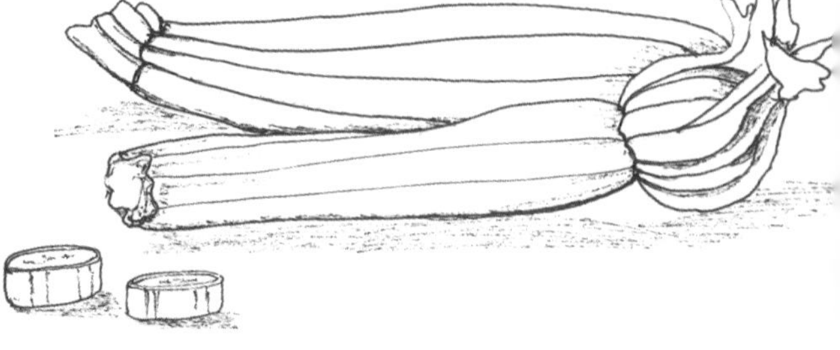

Nomato ketchup

stove top

This is good for those people who can't tolerate the nightshade family or can't have too much sugar or vinegar. Use on burgers or sausages.

- *1 onion, finely chopped*
- *1 small garlic clove, finely chopped*
- *1 medium beetroot, finely chopped*
- *1 medium carrot, finely chopped*
- *1 tbsp coconut oil*
- *1 tsp basil*
- *1 tbsp cider vinegar (optional)*
- *salt and pepper*

Sauté all the vegetables in a pan with the coconut oil for 5 minutes. Just cover them with water and simmer for 5 minutes or until they are all soft. Drain and add the basil, seasoning and vinegar, if using.

Leave to cool and blend together to a soft pulp. Push through a sieve for a smoother sauce.

This sauce will keep in the fridge for a day.

No-pasta lasagne with aubergine

oven

serves 4

If you can tolerate aubergine this is a good alternative to lasagne as it uses no dairy and no wheat, two of the main causes of food intolerance. If you can't eat aubergine, try this with courgettes.

The aubergine is raw in this recipe, but it can be seared for a richer flavour.

'Cheese'

- *110g (4oz) cashews*
- *100ml (3½fl oz) coconut milk*
- *juice of 1 lemon*
- *1 tbsp basil leaves*
- *2 garlic cloves*
- *salt and pepper*

Sauce

- *3 tbsp olive oil, plus extra for greasing*
- *1 onion, chopped*
- *1 tsp crushed garlic*
- *1 tsp ground cumin*
- *2 tsp dried oregano*
- *1 courgette (zucchini), chopped*
- *200g (7oz) cooked red or green lentils*
- *1 x 400g tin of chopped tomatoes*

Layers

- *2 aubergines (eggplants), sliced longways in ½cm (¼in) strips*

Blend all the 'cheese' ingredients together in a bowl and put them aside in the fridge.

Heat the oil in a saucepan and fry the onion, garlic, spices, herbs and some seasoning. Add the courgette, lentils and tomatoes and simmer for 20 minutes.

Heat the oven to 180°C/ fan160°C/350°F/Gas 4.

In an oiled baking dish, add a layer of aubergine, then a layer of 'cheese' followed by a layer of sauce. Continue to layer and finish with a layer of sauce or 'cheese'.

Bake for 35–40 minutes and allow to cool for 10 minutes before serving.

Nut cream

serves 4

Obviously, make sure your guests are not intolerant to nuts before serving this as an alternative to dairy cream. If possible, soak the nuts overnight before blending.

- *225g (8oz) chopped cashews or blanched almonds*
- *100ml (3½fl oz) rice, almond milk or water*
- *1 tsp honey or agave syrup (optional)*
- *1 tsp vanilla extract (optional)*

Blend everything together to form a smooth cream. Add a little more water if it's too thick.

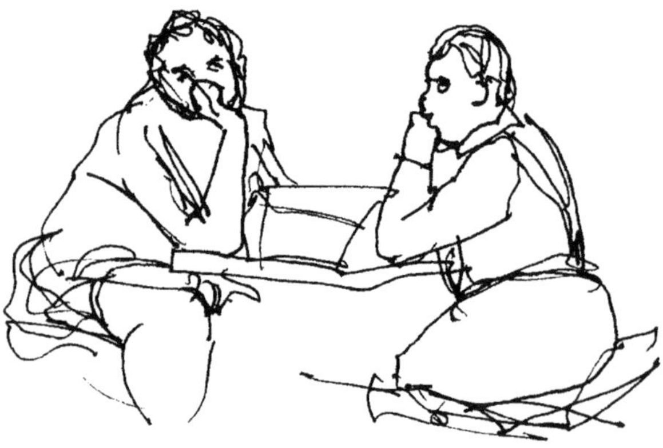

Pizza base (grain-free)

oven

makes 2 x 23cm (9in) pizza bases

Like BBQ night, pizza night can mean missing out for anyone who has food intolerance. This is a surprisingly tasty alternative to pizza pastry for everyone who can't eat any grain products. The pizza bases can be frozen.

- *125g (4½oz) raw pumpkin seeds*
- *60g (2oz) coconut flour*
- *1 tbsp ground chia*
- *1 tsp baking powder*
- *1 garlic clove, chopped (optional)*
- *1 tbsp cider vinegar (optional)*
- *250ml gluten-free broth or water*
- *salt and pepper*

Heat the oven to 180°C/ fan160°C/350°F/Gas 4.

Blend the dry ingredients in a food processor until the texture of cornmeal. Transfer to a large bowl and add the garlic and vinegar and enough broth to form a soft dough.

Divide the dough between 2 parchment-lined baking trays and spread it out to 5mm (¼in) thick. Place in the oven and bake for 10 minutes or until golden.

Cover with your preferred toppings and return to the oven for another 20 minutes.

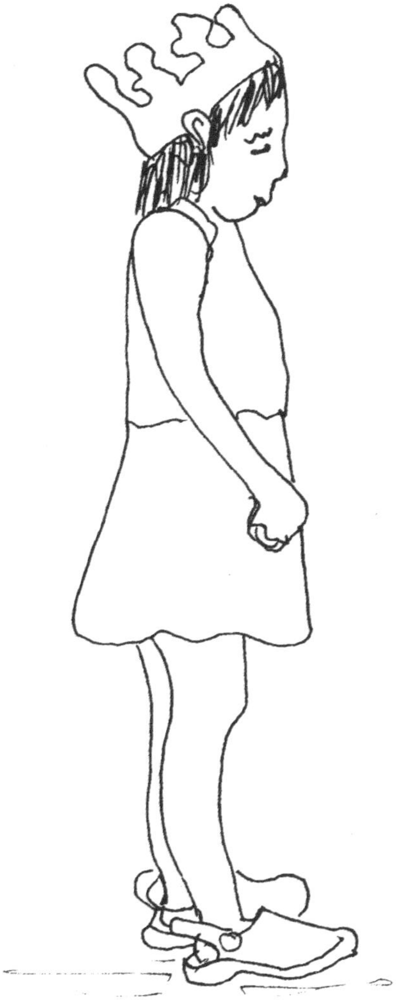

Vegan blueberry cheesecake

freezer

serves 4–6

Warn your guests that the vegan cheesecake contains nuts. This delicious recipe uses no dairy or grains. This recipe includes 450g (1lb) raw cashews that should be soaked overnight if possible.

Base

- *170g (6oz) walnuts*
- *110g (4oz) almonds*
- *225g (8oz) pitted dates*
- *½ tsp ground vanilla beans or extract*
- *Pinch of salt*

Cheesecake layer

- *450g (1lb) raw cashews (soaked overnight)*
- *75ml (3fl oz) lime or lemon juice*
- *5 tbsp honey or maple syrup*
- *1 tsp lime zest or more*
- *2 tsp vanilla extract*
- *75ml (3fl oz) coconut oil, melted*
- *225g (8oz) blueberries, to decorate*

Pulse all the ingredients for the base together in a food processor until a sticky crumble forms. Add a splash of water if needed and then press into an 18cm (7in) greased springform tin. Place in the fridge while making the cheesecake layer.

Rinse and drain the cashews and blend them until smooth (add a little water if too dry) in a blender, then add the lime juice, a quarter of the sweetener, the zest and vanilla and blend again. Pour in the coconut oil and pulse to combine. Taste and adjust for sweetness. Add the blueberries or blend them separately to use as a separate top layer.

Remove the base from the fridge and top with the cheesecake mixture, then freeze for 3 hours to firm up. Transfer to fridge to keep cold before serving.

Serve cold on the springform base.

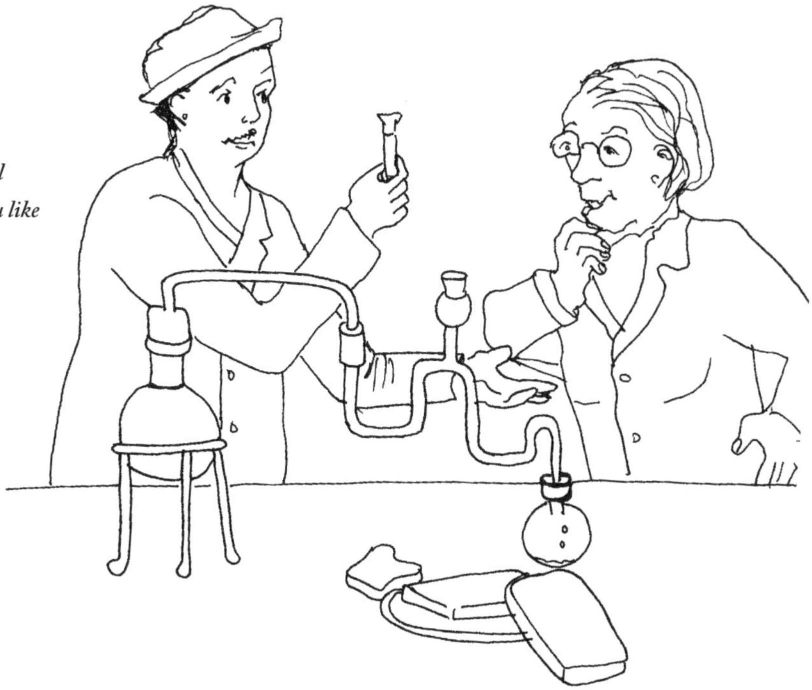

How much artificial colouring would you like on your toast?

ADDITIVES

'More than 90% of additives are for cosmetic reasons.'
The Guardian (Why We Eat This Way, 2003)

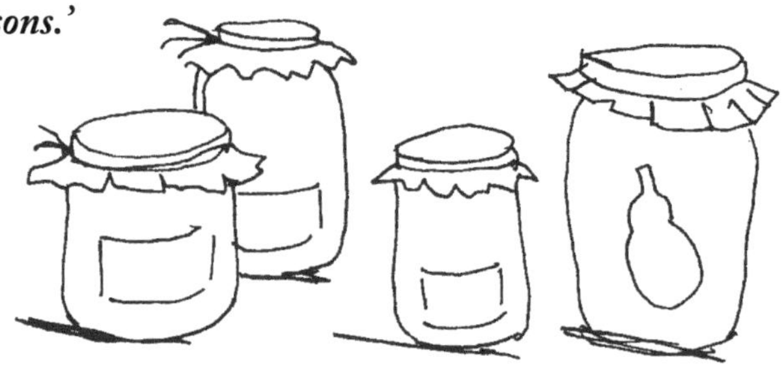

Homemade preserves avoid the additives.

'Additives' describes all the extras that get put into the main ingredients used in factory-produced food, to make them seem more appealing. Many of the meals we eat today are manufactured in factories. By the time the machine has finished making a meal, it may not look at all like what your granny used to eat. Then, after or during this process, comes the cosmetic work which will ensure a decent appearance and a long shelf life.

Over 540 additives are considered safe for human consumption, although critics say that so many should not be allowed. Of the additives that are permitted, over 70 may cause allergies and 30 may cause long-term harm to people who have allergic reactions to them. In the region of 4,500 different flavouring compounds are available to manufacturers, but they do not have to be tested for safety and are only banned if shown to be harmful.

Here is a list of what might be in your food:

Additives that have had reported effects:

Colour:

160b annatto, bixin, norbixin

Preservatives:

200 - 203 sorbic acid, sorbates

210 - 219 benzoic acid, benzoates

220 - 228 sulphur dioxide, sulphites, bisulfites, metabisulphites

249 - 252 nitrates and nitrites

280 - 283 propionic acid and propionates

320 - 321 BHA and BHT (Butylated Hydroxyanisole and Butylated Hydroxytoluene)

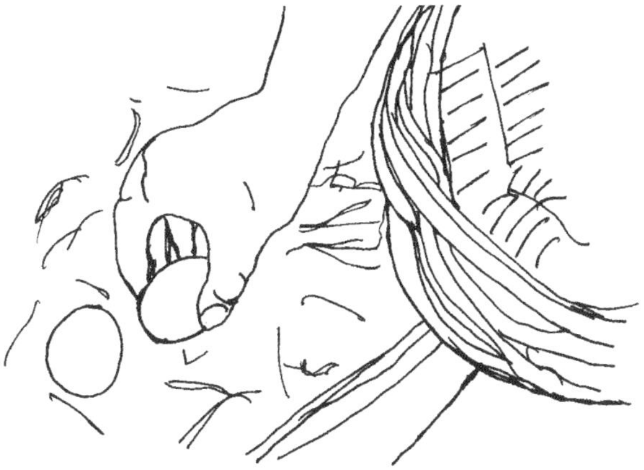

Just add an egg and all the colouring, antibiotics and pesticides the chickens were given before the production of that egg.

Colouring

If the product (the food you're about to eat) has become blanched by the processing method, food colouring will be added to make it look more tempting. A friend who used to pick strawberries each summer told me that they became white during processing, so their red colour had to be re-introduced artificially. Red jams are not all naturally so. And who wants to eat canned beige beef stew?

Coal-tar dyes came to the rescue of industrially processed foods for many years, but after campaigns complaining of allergic or behavioural reactions to these, we now have natural or nature-identical dyes. There are several campaigns about these, as some say that nature-identical dyes also have side-effects. But as there is little more than anecdotal evidence about this, they are still used by the food industry.

Michelle

Michelle was 14 when she went on a cycling trip to Portugal. One night, as a treat, the group cycled into town for supper rather than cook at the campsite. In a local café they had golden huevos. By the time they had cycled back to the woods, Michelle complained of a headache and then of itching, especially on her back and arms. She had erupted into hives.

Michelle had had abdominal migraines as a child and still had regular migraine headaches as a teenager. She had recently discovered she was sensitive to a variety of food additives, including some colourants and preservatives such as sodium benzoate and sodium metabisulfite.

She reckoned that her headache and her hives were caused by her histamine reaction to the eggs she had eaten, because sometimes chicken feed is laced with food colouring to make the yolks appear more yellow.

Rod, a helper, cycled to the nearest pharmacy and, after much acting and confusion, came back with antihistamine cream and pills.

By the time they all had to cycle on, Michelle could manage as long as she was masked in a scarf and sunglasses.

Michelle still gets migraines, but less so now that she rarely eats out and has eliminated most of the trigger foods from her daily diet.

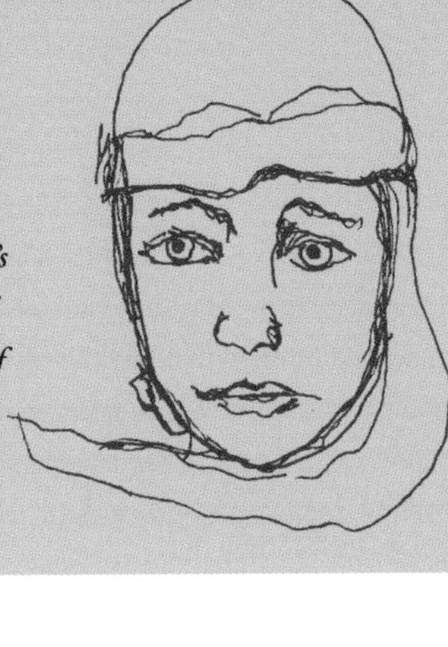

Michelle's cover-all headscarf

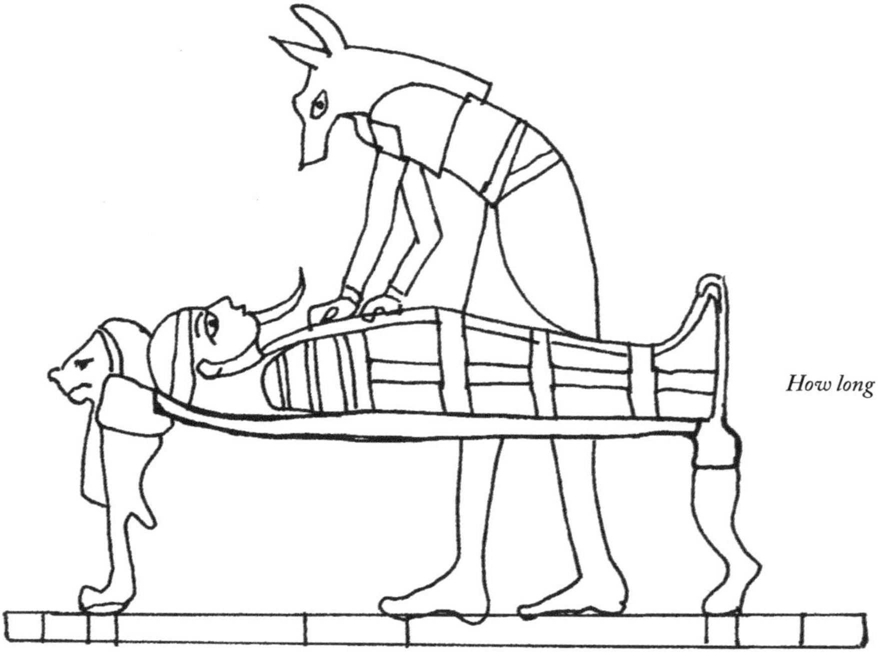

How long a shelf life did you say?

Preservatives

There is a vast array of chemicals available to make the product last longer on the shelf and stop it from mouldering. These chemicals have a variety of uses, from manufactured carbon dioxide used to create a protective atmosphere to coal-tar chemicals, (such as BHA and BHT (Butylated Hydroxyanisole and Butylated Hydroxytoluene) used to prevent rancidity and extend shelf life of breakfast cereals) and which, according to the WHO, give side-effects including skin irritation, sun sensitivity, allergic reactions, and skin discoloration, during manufacture as well as after eating.

Flavours

Many manufactured foods contain chemical smells and tastes. Some are used to cover rancidity, which is caused by the production process or brought on by the resulting extended shelf life. Think of the nice, buttery, vanilla smell of margarine or butter substitute. Others flavours are introduced to stimulate the taste buds and the feeling that we just must have MORE of that taste.

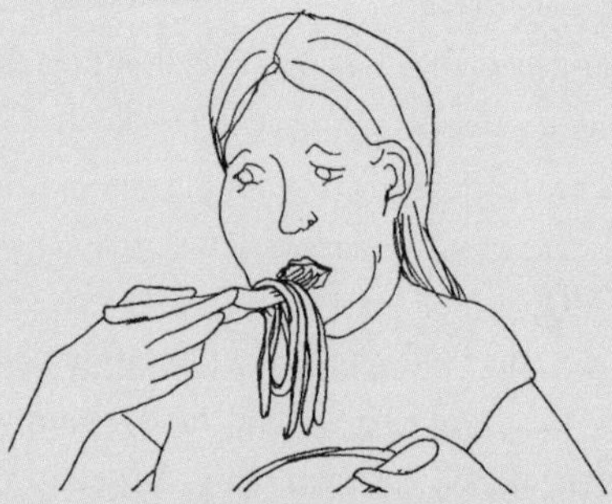

NO MSG PLEASE Let's go eat Italian!

Jackie

Jackie came for a party and stayed the next day to help clear up. By the evening everyone was tired, so she kindly offered to pick up a Chinese takeaway for everyone. When the food was shared out everyone expressed surprise that it seemed tasteless and there wasn't much gravy on anything. Usually the takeaway was really good. Jackie beamed: 'I asked them to use no MSG, I can't have it and I knew you wouldn't mind!' Her friends were all polite but vowed never, ever to let her collect any food again!

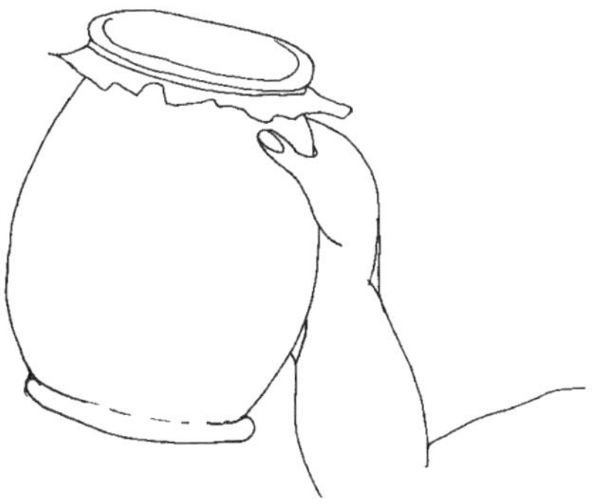

Bulking agents

These are just that. They function as ballast to make up weight or hide a lack of substance in the finished product. So it could be the thickener in your pie gravy or the gelling agent that makes your ice-cream fluffier. Some bulking agents can trigger food intolerances.

Additives in the UK and Europe have been given specific E numbers for ease of labelling (the 'E' stands for Europe). The idea is that their toxicology has been tested and seen to meet EU standards. Some food additives that are permitted in the EU are not permitted in other countries and vice versa. Some E numbers are natural and familiar, such as E948 – oxygen (used as a gas environment for packing), E300 – vitamin C (used as a preservative) and E101 – vitamin B2 (used as a food colour).

Some of these approved additives are known to cause harmful effects in some people. For instance, sulphur dioxide (E220), which is used as a steriliser and preservative in wine, can exacerbate asthma symptoms. Look for more information online if you experience any of the reported symptoms, such as itching, trouble breathing, hives or nettle rash.

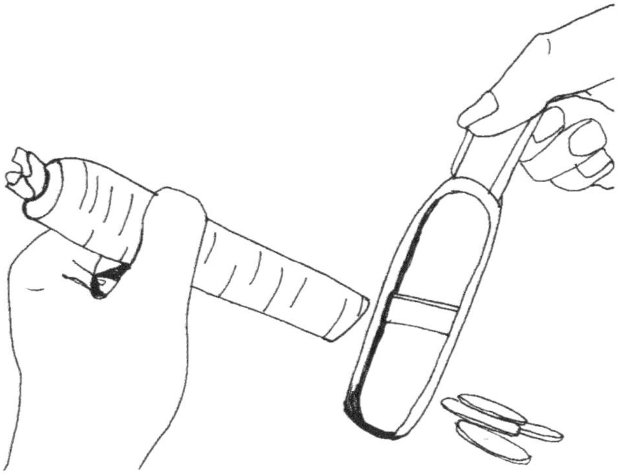

RECIPES

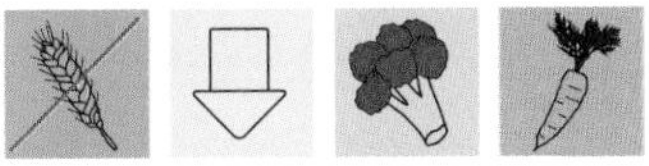

Vegetable crisps

stove top

per person

Many packaged crisps contain rice flour and wheat starch, MSG, dextrose and other flavour enhancers that aid the perception of a savoury flavour.

- *3cm (1¼in) piece of parsnip, carrot, beetroot, potato*
- *100ml (3½fl oz) frying oil*
- *salt and pepper*

Using a mandolin or a knife, cut the veg into very thin slices and place them on a clean tea towel and pat them to dry slightly.

Heat the oil in a wok or deep pan until it is hot enough that a piece of veg sizzles when you drop it into the oil. Deep-fry the vegetable slices in small batches, separating any that stick together. Remove them from the pan with a slotted spoon as they become golden brown, and transfer to a plate lined with a paper towel to drain off the excess oil. Season to taste.

These are best eaten immediately.

Homemade bacon

serves up to 8

Commercial bacon often includes potassium nitrate and sodium nitrite that are known to be risks to health. This makes a lardon-type salty bacon.

- *500g (1lb 2oz) salt*
- *125g (4½oz) muscovado sugar*
- *1 tsp ground black pepper*
- *1kg (2¼lb) pork belly – around 3 pieces*

In a non-metallic bowl, combine the salt, sugar and pepper.

On a clean surface, rub the salt mix into the pork belly, one piece at a time. Transfer any unused salt mix to a jar, seal and set aside.

Stack the meat pieces one on top of another in a container, cover with a clean cloth and weigh down with something heavy (such as weights from an old set of scales or a couple of large jars full of water). Set aside in the fridge for one day, after which time there should be liquid in the container.

The next day, drain off the liquid, rub more of the reserved salt mix into the pork and re-stack the pile of meat pieces in a different order. Cover and weigh down as before.

Repeat daily for 4 days, then dry once more and refrigerate, wrapped in greaseproof paper. Slice as desired.

If the salty taste is too much, wash the bacon and pat dry before use.

Bacon, cabbage & rice

stove top

serves 4

This recipe is a tasty way to use your homemade bacon.

- *350g (12oz) brown rice*
- *1 tbsp frying oil*
- *225g (8oz) thinly sliced rashers of homemade bacon (see left)*
- *1 onion, finely chopped*
- *½ small cabbage, thinly sliced*
- *pinch of salt*
- *1 tsp roughly ground black pepper*
- *1 tbsp tamari*
- *1 litre (1¾ pints) boiling water*

Cook the rice in a pan with plenty of salted water for around 35 minutes, or until just soft and done. Drain.

About 10 minutes before the rice is ready, heat the oil in a frying pan and fry the bacon until almost crispy, then add the onion and fry for a few more minutes. Add the cabbage and seasonings and fry for 1 minute.

Pour enough hot water into the pan to make a thin gravy and simmer for 10 minutes until the cabbage is soft. Mix the cooked rice into the hot sauce mix to warm through just before serving.

Season to taste, adding more water if it has become dry. Serve immediately.

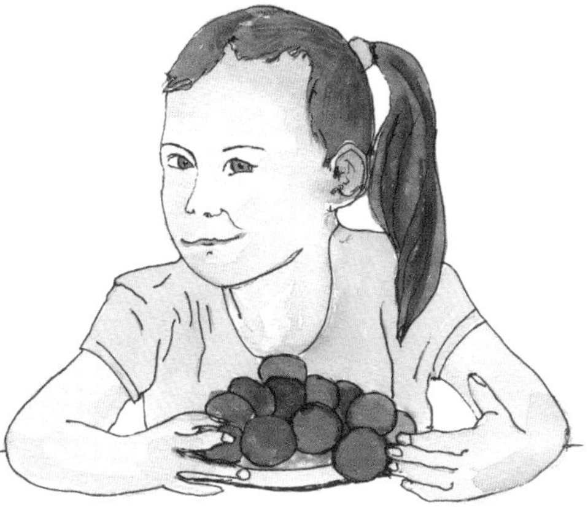

Bonvive balls 1

serves 4

A healthy alternative to chocolate.

- *1 tsp carob powder*
- *50g (2oz) finely chopped sultanas or dates*
- *2 ripe bananas, mashed*
- *1–2 tsp water or fruit juice*
- *2 tbsp desiccated (shredded) coconut*

Sift the carob powder into a bowl to remove any lumps, then mix in the sultanas or dates and mashed bananas. Add enough liquid to bind the mix, then dig out chunks of the mixture and form them into 2cm (¾in) balls.

Dust a clean chopping board with the coconut and roll the balls to coat them. Place on a plate and transfer to the fridge for 30 minutes to set.

Bonvive balls 2

serves 4

An alternative to sweets or cakes, which may contain sweeteners and other additives.

- *50g (2oz) dates*
- *225g (8oz) mixed nuts*
- *1 tbsp tahini*
- *½ tsp vanilla paste*
- *a splash of rice milk or fruit juice*
- *2 tbsp desiccated (shredded) coconut*

Blend all the nuts until finely chopped, transfer to a bowl and mix with the tahini and vanilla paste. Add enough liquid to bind the mix, then dig out chunks of the mixture and form them into 2cm (¾in) balls.

Dust a clean chopping board with the coconut and roll the balls to cover them. Place on a plate and transfer to the fridge for 30 minutes to set.

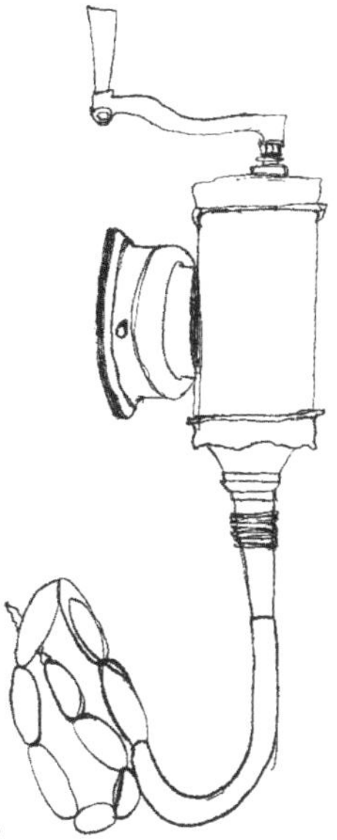

Sausages

stove top

serves 4

Sodium nitrite, sodium nitrate, potassium nitrate and phosphates are widely used as added ingredients in sausages. All of these can be carcinogenic. This is the simplest of sausages to make. You can add other flavours to the mix if you like, such as chopped apple or leek, chilli or mustard.

- *1kg (2¼lb) minced lamb, beef or pork*
- *2 tbsp chopped herbs: rosemary, sage, thyme, dried basil*
- *225g (8oz) gluten-free breadcrumbs (optional)*
- *pinch of salt*
- *1 tsp black pepper (optional)*
- *sausage skins (optional – from local butchers or buy online)*

Mix all the ingredients, except for the sausage skins, together really well in a bowl.

Take a little ball of this mixture and fry it in a pan, taste, then adjust the flavours for the rest of the mixture, if necessary.

Stuff the filling into the skins using a sausage machine, or just form some skinless sausages. Fry in a frying pan until golden brown and cooked through, pricking the skins (if they have them) before cooking.

If you like, you can make a big batch and freeze them, wrapped, for future use.

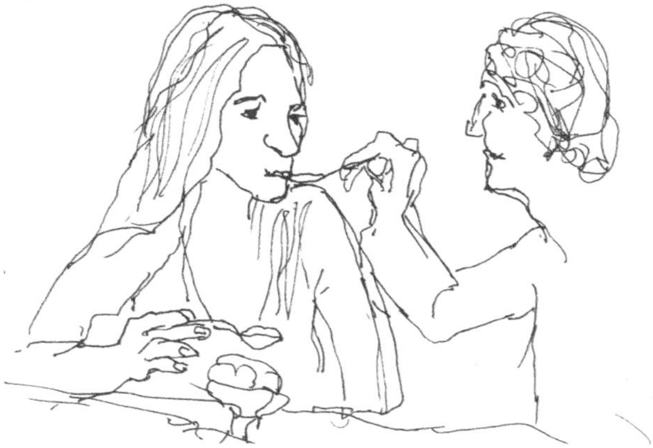

Onion gravy

stove top

serves 4

There's no need to use packet gravy mixes to go with your sausages.

- *2 small onions, finely sliced*
- *oil, for frying*
- *2 garlic cloves, pressed*
- *240ml (8fl oz) water or stock*
- *1 tsp tamari*
- *1 tbsp gluten-free flour*
- *salt and pepper*

Fry the onions in a pan in a little oil until they are crispy and brown. Add the garlic and fry for 1 more minute, then pour in the water or stock and tamari. Mash everything together.

Mix the flour with a little cold water in a small bowl and stir well, then add it to the stock mix, stirring. Add more liquid for a thinner gravy. Bring to the boil and simmer, stirring occasionally, for 2 minutes.

Taste and adjust the seasoning. Serve in a warmed jug.

Tropical vegan ice-cream

freezer

serves 4–6

There is a long list of possible additives in ice-cream, such as propylene glycol (also used in antifreeze), glycerine, sodium carboxymethyl cellulose, monoglycerides, diglycerides, disodium phosphates, tetrasodium pyrophosphate, polysorbate 80, and dioctyl sodium sulfosuccinate. This is the healthy alternative.

It is best to make this the morning of the day it is to be served so it is still fresh tasting.

- *3–4 frozen sliced bananas*
- *1 block creamed coconut, sliced*
- *2 peaches, sliced*
- *3 slices of tinned pineapple*
- *2 tbsp lime juice*

Blend all the ingredients in a blender until smooth. Transfer to an ice-cream maker and follow the manufacturer's instructions, or pour into a freezerproof tub and freeze, stirring with a fork to break up the granules every half hour or so until it's frozen through.

Defrost at room temperature for 30 minutes to soften and stir through before serving.

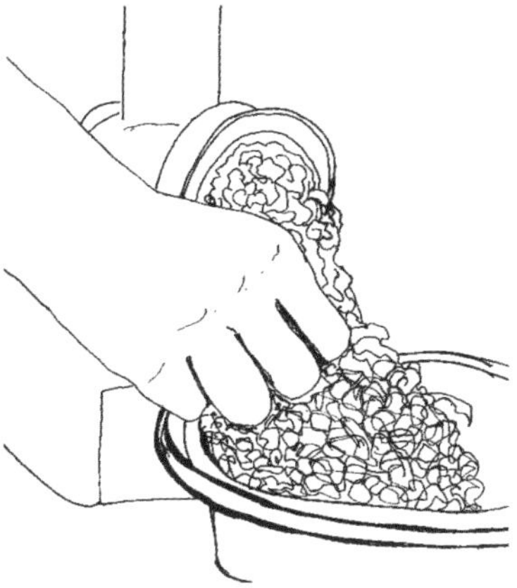

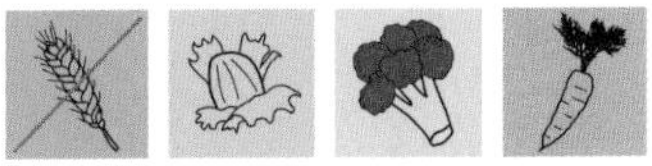

Christmas mincemeat

enough for 4 x 454g (1lb) jars

This contains only what you would like to eat, so no sulphites in the dried fruit or fungicides in the apple and no lard nor beef fat.

- *225g (8oz) raisins*
- *225g (8oz) sultanas*
- *225g (8oz) currants*
- *1kg (2¼lb) cooking apples, cored, peeled and sliced*
- *100g (3½oz) chopped blanched almonds (optional)*
- *100g (3½oz) muscovado sugar (use less if you wish)*
- *1 tsp ground cinnamon*
- *2 tsp grated nutmeg*
- *1 tbsp brandy or whisky (optional)*

Mince the raisins, sultanas and apples in a mincer, if you have one, or, if you don't, finely chop them. Add the fruit to a large bowl and use your hands to combine with all the other ingredients. Cover the bowl and leave overnight at room temperature for all the flavours to mingle and the dried fruit to absorb the liquid.

Next day, taste, and adjust the spices if need be, then spoon into clean and sterilised jars, topping up with a little more brandy, if you like.

Seal and store in a cool place until needed or for up to 1 year.

To sterilise jam jars, heat the oven to 140°C/ fan120°C/275°F/Gas 1. Wash the jars in hot, soapy water, then rinse well. Place the jars and lids on a baking sheet and put them in the oven to dry completely.

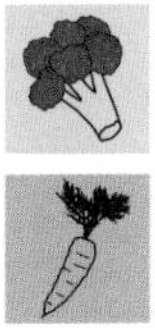

Hot cross buns

moderate oven

makes 12

Commercial hot cross buns have a huge range of additives. Just the sugars can be sweeteners, including maple syrup, dextrose, invert sugar, glucose and maltodextrin. They also contain emulsifiers, thickeners and preservatives. These are best split in half and toasted.

Buns

- *450g (1lb) wholewheat spelt bread flour, plus extra for dusting*
- *1 tsp salt*
- *1 sachet instant dried yeast*
- *2 tsp grated nutmeg*
- *1 tsp ground cinnamon*
- *200g (7oz) raisins*
- *1 tbsp muscovado sugar (optional)*
- *300–400ml (10–14fl oz) warm water*

Crosses

- *2 tbsp white spelt flour*
- *1 tbsp cold water*

Sugar and water glaze (optional)

- *1 tbsp white sugar*
- *2 tbsp boiled water*

In a bowl, combine all the dry ingredients for the buns. Slowly add enough warm water to make a soft dough. Cover and leave at room temperature to rise until doubled in size, then knock it down with your fist and knead it on a work surface or board dusted with flour for about 5 minutes.

Divide the dough into 12 balls and place them on a floured baking tray.

Allow the buns to rise as you make a paste from the white spelt and water, stirring them together in a bowl to make a pastry-like consistency. Roll this to a flat floured sheet and cut strips to make the crosses. Use a dab of water to fix the strips cross ways on the top of the buns. Cover with a clean tea towel and leave to rise until doubled.

Heat the oven to 180°C/ fan160°C/350°F/Gas 4, then bake the buns for 20–30 minutes or until golden brown. Transfer to a wire rack to cool.

While the buns are cooling, make the glaze, if you like. Combine the sugar and water in a small pan and boil for 5 minutes to create a sugary syrup. Once the buns are cool, brush them with the glaze.

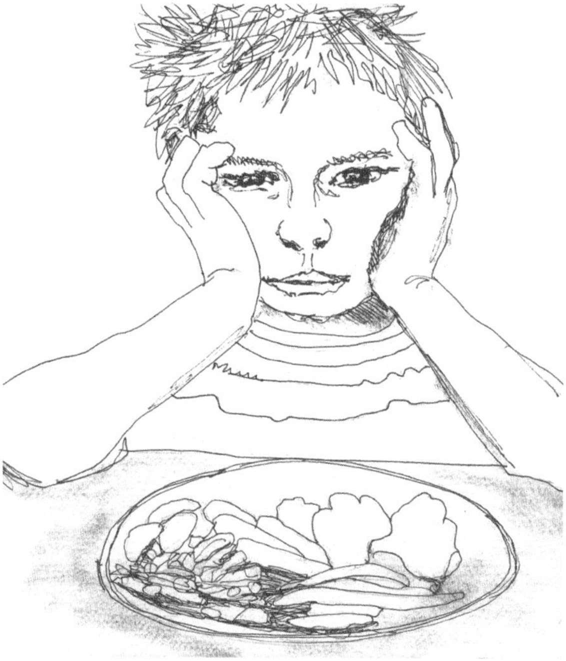

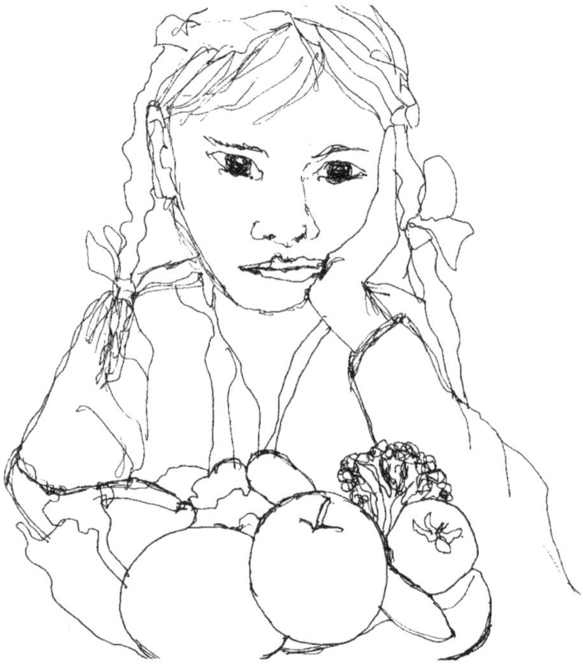

FUSSY EATERS & SUPER TASTERS

It has been suggested that there are between five and twelve different fundamental tastes: sweet, sour, salty, bitter and umami (savoury) are the most well known, possibly joined by calcium, kokumi (heartiness), piquance (spiciness), coolness, metallicity, fat and carbon dioxide (as in the sparkle in soda water).

Our sense of taste through evolution has developed to choose foods high in nutrition and to warn us off poisons, so children are drawn to sweet tastes because at early stages of growth and development there is a need for high-energy foods. Pregnant women tend to become more sensitive to bitter tastes, perhaps to protect vulnerable foetuses from potential toxins.

Taste is, of course, entangled with all the other senses: sight, touch, sound and smell. Foods taste blander if we can't see them and, sometimes, blindfolded, our ability to even tell what they are vanishes altogether. In blind tasting, we can only accurately identify fruit juices about 20 per cent of the time. If fruit drinks are dyed in unusual colours we are deceived, so orange juice that is coloured purple tastes like grape.

Taste is mostly perceived by the nose and the retro-nasal smell centre, located in the nasal passages of the back of the mouth, when we exhale or swallow. As we age, the number of sensory cells that perceive aromas in the nose begins to decrease, and we start to lose taste buds. In people post-50, the replacement rate for sensory cells slows down until more cells are lost than are replaced, so older people do not have the taste ability of the young.

Charlie

My father, Charlie, who died when he was 94, lived on a diet of two Weetabix and a protein drink for the last two years of his life. He had always been a fussy eater. It took me many years, but I eventually realised that it was not my place to change his life but just to accept his attitude to food.

Supertasters

Supertasters have significantly more taste receptors than most people. The average person has between 18–35 taste receptors on each tastebud, while super tasters have 35–60. This increased sensitivity can make them fussy eaters, as they can be overwhelmed by strong tastes, such as the piquancy of spicy dishes like curry or chilli, or they may dislike bitterness in foods such as broccoli and Brussels sprouts.

Children

This story appeared on the BBC in September 2019 and alerts us to the fact that something as seemingly innocuous as fussy eating can have severe consequences.

'Experts are warning about the risks of extreme fussy eating after a teenager developed permanent sight loss after living on a diet of chips and crisps.'

One of our children was such a fussy eater that we had a list they had compiled named 'foods I might like'. On it were the blandest of ingredients: white bread, white rice, macaroni. But also, there was curry! Many children do not like mixtures but will eat plain foods willingly. Cake but not with raisins, cucumber, tomato or carrot sticks and lettuce leaves but not together as a salad.

Some do better if they are allowed to roam around while eating, use their hands or be fed like a baby while they are young. It will not always be like this, so a little tolerance as they go through these stages helps to keep everything cool.

For other children it is a little more complex. These children are genetically made to be super-tasters. Anything that tastes hot, bitter or savoury, or that has a particular texture can be like being struck to these super-tasting children. So they need a little more patience, and serving bland food with a request to have 'a try', may help. After the third or fourth time of trying, apparently something settles into place and previously unappealing food can become more acceptable.

Fred

'I don't care if you don't like it, you liked it all last week when we had it.'

'Ugh!'

'Try a spoonful and stop pulling that face. You will find it's actually nice if you try some.'

When Fred was six years old, he had trouble eating. He had been this way since he was weaned as a one-year-old. He disliked many flavours and textures and he loved sugar.

The week before, he had been trying to fix an orange gum shield in his mouth before playing rugby. He had had complete control of how and when it entered his mouth to wrap around his gums and still he had vomited every time – even to the point where, when he held it near his nose, the smell induced retching. When he wouldn't eat the soup because it had carrot pieces in it, his mum was very, very patient and eventually he was persuaded to the trying stage.

'Oh, it's actually all right.' He said brightly, as though the last 15 minutes hadn't happened. After finishing the bowlful, he asked for a little more.

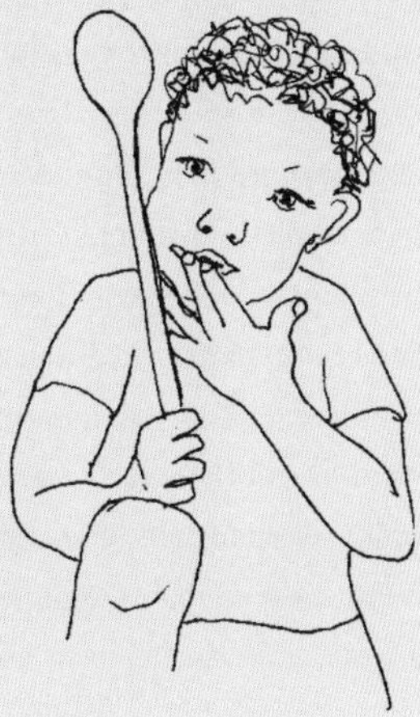

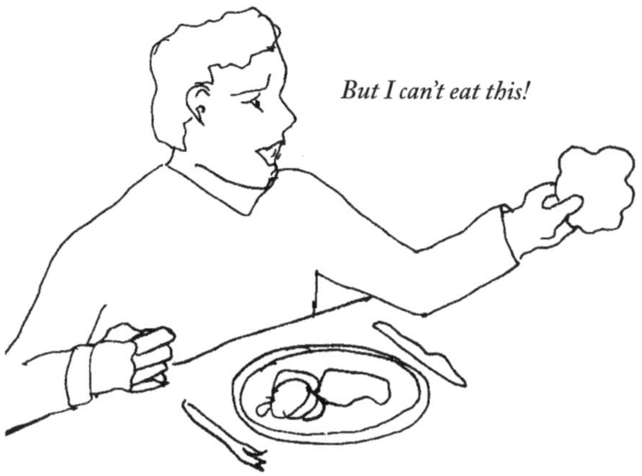

Adults

These can be fussy eaters, too. This can be because they too are supertasters or just because they picked up bad habits as a child and have never addressed them.

Henry

Henry had grown up on a dairy farm and loved eating their produce. Every meal involved dairy; there was cream on milky porridge at breakfast and lashings of butter on bread. However, Henry became vegetarian when he was ten, after finding out what happened to the excess male calves. But he was a vegetarian who did not like eating vegetables unless they were disguised in some way. Then, as a teenager, he virtually lived on cheesy toasties.

His food fads continued into adulthood. When he stayed with us, vegetable soup would be okay, as long as it was topped with enough cheese and served with bread and butter. His favourite meal was a baked potato, but only if it was served with butter, cheese and baked beans – and in no other way. Over time, we encouraged him to try salad, which he did eventually come to like as long as it was accompanied by lashings of mayonnaise.

RECIPES

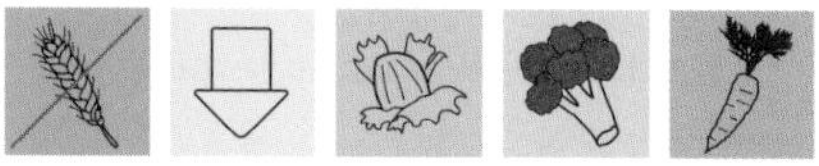

Pea soup

stove top

serves 4

A quick soup which goes down well with our fussy eaters. A swirl of cream or yoghurt can be added for those less fussy. This can be warmed on the stove top or served raw if you prefer.

- *450g (1lb) garden peas (fresh or frozen)*
- *300ml (10fl oz) carrot juice (fresh or frozen)*
- *pinch of grated nutmeg*
- *½ creamed avocado or 300ml (10fl oz) vegan cream*
- *1 tsp finely chopped chives*
- *6 small mint leaves (optional)*
- *salt and pepper*

Put the peas, carrot juice and nutmeg in a blender and pulse into smooth.

Add the avocado or cream and chives, stir thoroughly and season to taste. Garnish with the mint leaves, if using, just before serving.

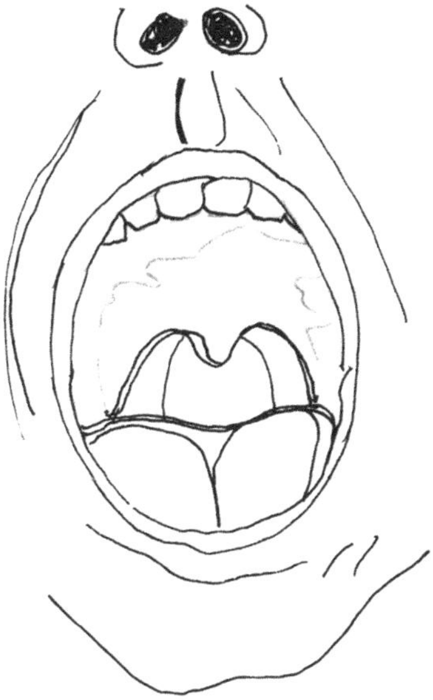

Taste is mostly perceived by the nose and the retro-nasal smell centre, located in the nasal passages of the back of the mouth, when we exhale or swallow.

Spelt pizza base

oven

makes 6–8

Sometimes pizza is the only thing worth eating and then only with a smear of tomato sauce and a ration of cheese. Spelt is a healthy alternative to gluten-rich wheat.

Do not knead this dough as spelt loses its form when kneaded.

- *1kg (2¼lb) white spelt flour or buckwheat, plus extra for dusting*
- *1 tsp grated nutmeg (optional)*
- *20g (¾oz) salt*
- *3 tsp instant dried yeast*
- *600ml (1 pint) warm water*
- *4 tbsp oil*

Combine the flour, nutmeg, salt and yeast together in a large mixing bowl.

Mix the warm water and oil together in a bowl and stir into the flour mix until well blended. If the dough is stiff add more water; if runny add more flour. Aim for a soft but well-formed texture.

To make 23-cm (9-in) pizzas, weigh out 130g (4½oz) balls of dough and set them on a tray covered with a clean tea towel for easy rolling later.

When ready to use, roll them out on a well-floured board.

Roast squash

hot oven

serves 4

The nice thing about squash is that it is sweet enough to appeal to the fussy while being full of vitamins A, B2, B6, B12 and C and minerals such as magnesium, phosphorus, and potassium as well as dietary fibre. You can follow this same recipe for sweet potatoes, too.

- *1 squash, peeled and cut into 3cm (1¼in) cubes*
- *1 tbsp olive or sunflower oil*
- *2 garlic cloves, chopped*
- *1 tsp dried or 2 tsp fresh chopped sage or rosemary*
- *1 tsp coriander seeds (optional)*
- *salt and pepper*

Heat the oven to 200°C/ fan180°C/400°F/Gas 6.

Put the squash in a roasting tray with the oil, garlic and sage or rosemary, making sure everything is covered in oil. Season and sprinkle with coriander seeds, if using.

Bake in the oven for 35–40 minutes or until crispy.

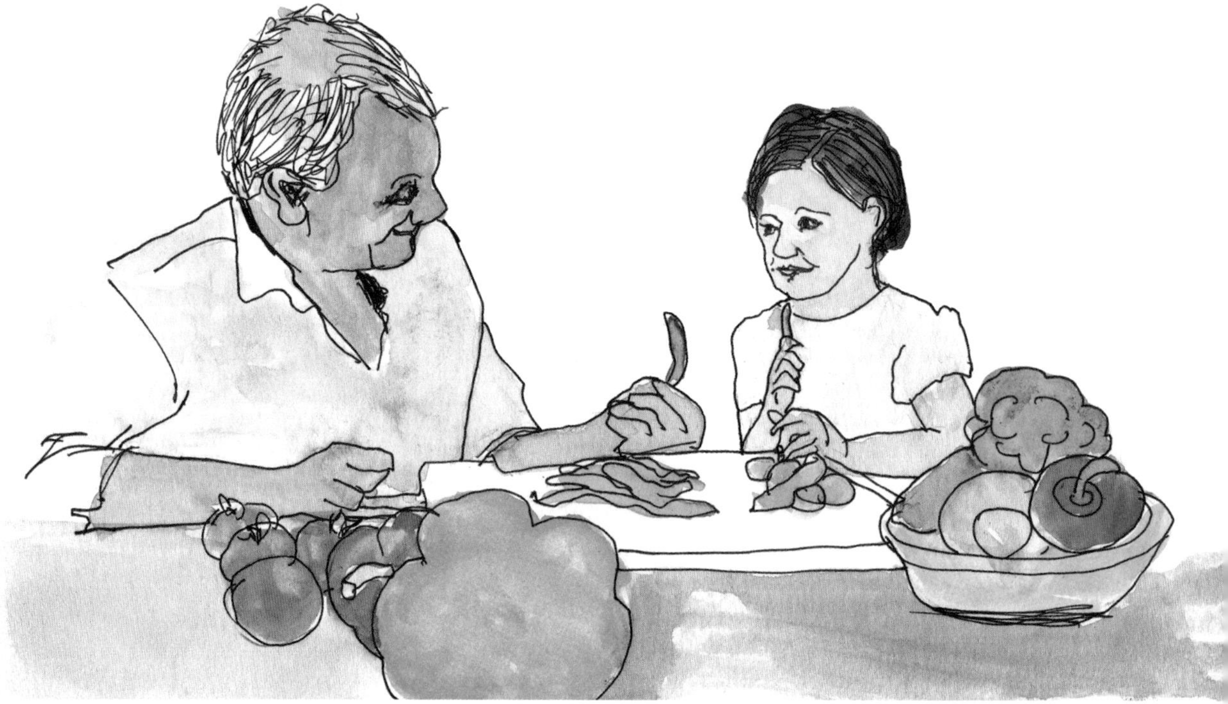

I know you want an orange but how about a nice bean instead?

FRUIT

Fruits are a mixed bunch. There are acid fruits and starchy fruits and fruits that we treat as vegetables. If you look online you will see fruits such as apples, blueberries and lemons are present in lists of both acid and alkaline fruits.

Although catastrophic allergic reaction to fruit is rare, they do cause symptoms in some people who are intolerant. These symptoms vary widely from person to person.

Oral Allergy Syndrome (OAS) is fairly rare and seems to be caused by particular proteins in some fruits, (and in other foods such as nuts), triggering the immune system. People who suffer OAS may experience itching, burning or stinging sensations of the mouth, throat and tongue as their body reacts to these proteins in the fruit which allergy antibodies mistake for pollen.

Acid fruits include:

- **oranges**
- **satsumas**
- **grapefruit**
- **limes**
- **grapes**
- **strawberries**
- **pineapple**
- **peaches**

Acid fruits can also be a cause of dental caries, particularly in young children, so are worth offering in moderation to the young. Alkaline fruits could be offered instead. However, these can also cause allergy and intolerance. Alkaline options include:

- **bananas**
- **kiwi**
- **mango**
- **melon**

Marley

'Why do I always cry on my birthday?'

I felt cruel denying Marley the occasional orange, satsuma or tangerine on special occasions and she always had problems with her birthday and with Christmas. She would become very irritable and miserable just when everyone else was beginning to enjoy the season. She would behave badly and madly as the excitement got too much for her and become tearful too. It took years for us to work out that this coincided with her special citrus treat. The emotional symptoms would come on before the physical symptoms emerged and from that time we had no oranges in the house and we made sure Marley's consumption of acidic foods was kept to a minimum.

Marley's sensitivity turned out to be not just to oranges, which she really cannot have, but to other citrus and acid foods if she has too many. So lemon, grapefruit, limes and even vinegar can cause her problems if she over-indulges. She can now eat acid fruits and vinegar most of the time but oranges still affect her emotionally.

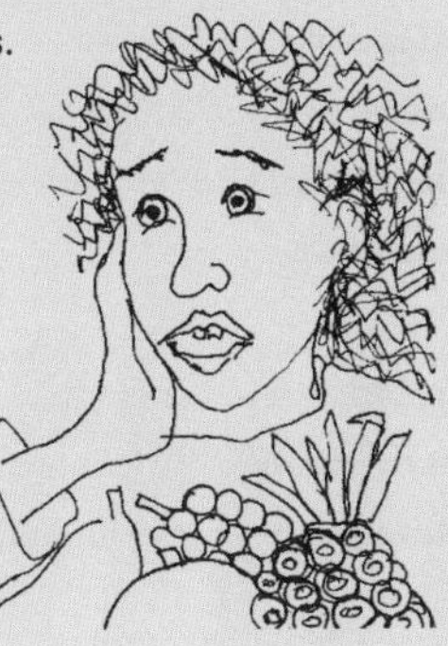

Fruit can have an effect on the gut flora by making the gut an acid environment, causing bloating and wind. It is thought that many of today's inflammatory conditions are caused by our bodies becoming too acidic.

If I eat uncooked dried fruit I have trouble; I have problems with bloat and wind so I don't eat too many raisins, sultanas, and certainly not prunes. I can eat fresh fruit like apples and pears and plums without any bother, though.

Olivia

Olivia is a fitness trainer and an old friend. We were deep in conversation at the swimming pool when suddenly I had the urge to belch. I apologised and Olivia asked if I had been eating fruit, which I hadn't. Olivia then told me that she had given up eating fruit altogether. This tall, willowy, fit woman had suffered for years from bloating and wind. But after a month's trip to Iceland, where she had eaten no fruit whatsoever, all her symptoms had disappeared. Now, she avoids any fruit and eats vegetables such as carrots and peppers in their place.

Some say that citrus in the form of oranges (sometimes grapefruit, too) can increase mucus within the body system, which is why it causes a reaction. Others say it is the acidity in citrus fruits that causes the problem – except for lemons, which are said to have an alkali effect. That seems very confusing, so it is easiest for cooks to stay clear of citrus in all its forms if you know that someone with a reaction to any of them is coming to eat with you.

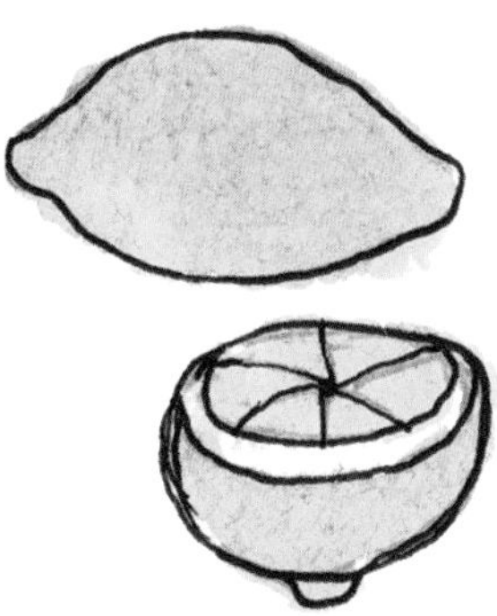

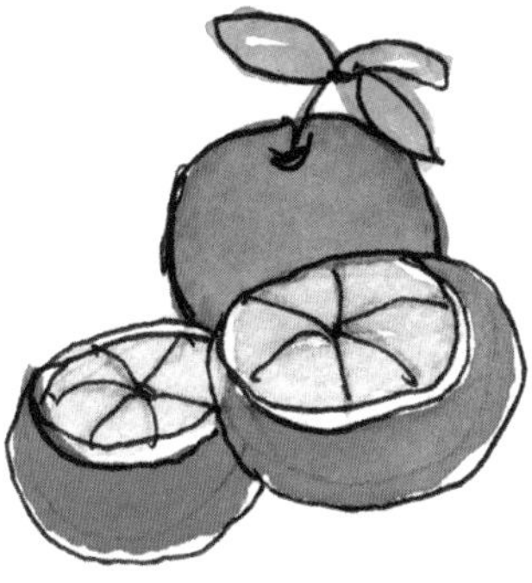

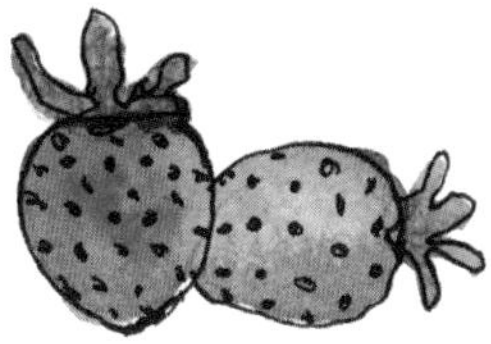

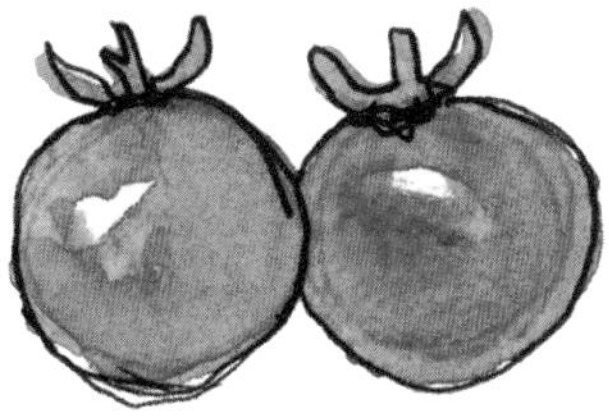

Me, Ann & Catherine

It was lunchtime at the yoga workshop. The morning's flow session had been hard, but then delicious cake was served. I was deep in conversation when a slight itch in my nose made me aware that someone near me was peeling an orange. I quickly left the room and joined Ann who, it turned out, was also avoiding the orange zest. Since she was tiny, Ann had reacted to oranges. At first she would have a whole body rash, but now it appeared just around her neck, throat and face. We were joined by Catherine, who was also escaping. Catherine said that if she accidentally eats any orange (including dried peel), she would have the headaches and biliousness of a hangover that would last for two days. Ann and I looked at each other and suddenly felt luckier!

There are some people for whom even a small amount of fruit can be problematic. These people are intolerant to the natural sugar found in fruit (fructose). For such people, eating fructose may lead to gut symptoms including abdominal discomfort, diarrhoea and bloating.

Fruitarianism

Fruitarianism is a kind of dietary veganism that consists of eating mostly fruits without animal products. Between 50–75 per cent of the fruitarian diet can be made up predominantly of raw fruit. Some people also include nuts, seeds and grains.

Fruitarians have different reasons for their dietary choice, including ethical, environmental, cultural and health considerations. As well as what we typically consider to be fruit, like apples and peaches, fruitarians may also eat vegetables like tomatoes, cucumber, peppers and avocado. Some of these foods, such as avocado, make an important contribution to fat intake, while nuts and seeds provide some protein and micro-nutrients.

It is thought that fruitarian diets can lead to deficiency in nutrients such as vitamin B12, calcium, iron, zinc, omega-3 and protein, though, so these need to be provided in supplementary form.

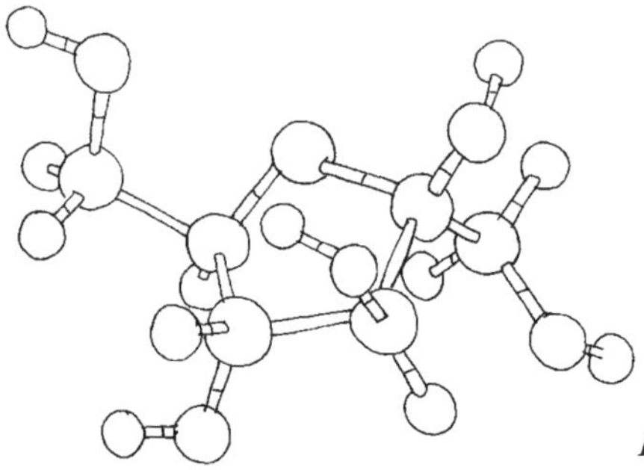

Fructose

RECIPES

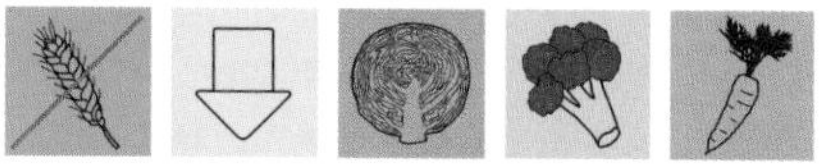

Avocado & sunflower seed mayo dip

serves 4

Good for fruitarians but also anyone who can't have lemons, this is also a tasty alternative to normal salad dressing. Use this thick as a dip or add more water to thin for mayonnaise. To use as a dressing, thin with soya milk.

- *100g (3½oz) sunflower seeds*
- *½ avocado*
- *200ml (7fl oz) water*
- *¼ onion or 1 garlic clove, chopped (optional)*
- *chopped basil or mint (optional)*
- *salt and pepper*

Put all the ingredients into a blender and blend until smooth, adding a little more water if it gets too thick. Season to taste. Serve immediately.

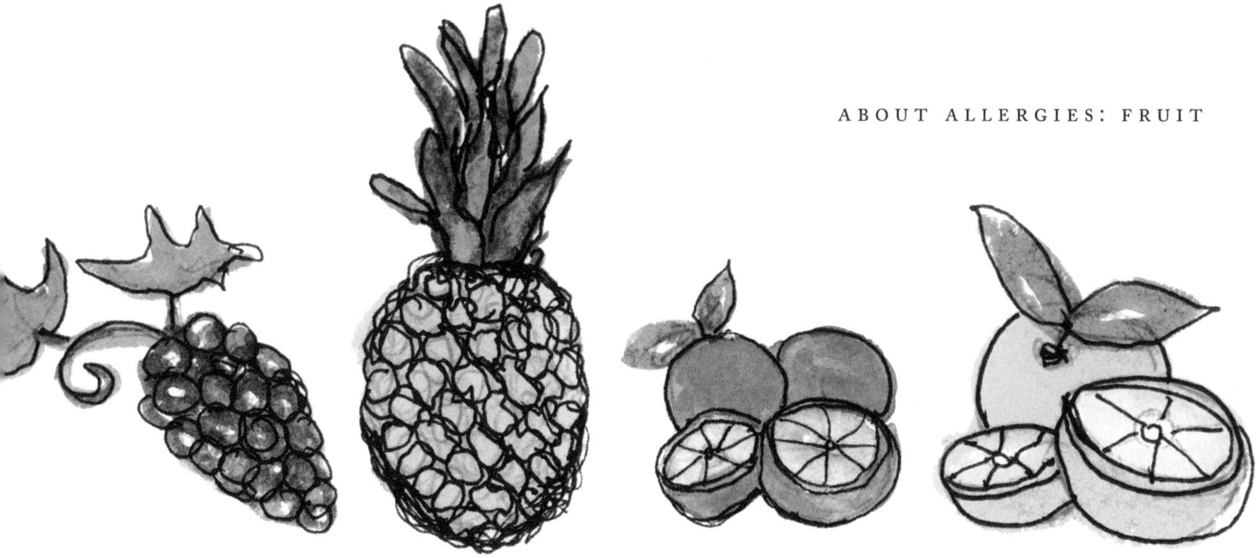

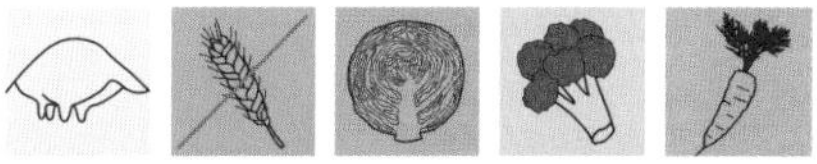

Avocado guacamole

serves 2

Another good recipe for fruitarians as well as to go with old favourites such as Huevas Rancheros (see page 134) or Falafels (see page 134)

- *1 ripe avocado*
- *1 tsp olive oil per avocado*
- *l tsp lemon juice per avocado*
- *1 garlic clove per avocado or adjust to taste*
- *1 tbsp chopped coriander leaves (cilantro), chilli or tomatoes (optional)*
- *1 tbsp live plain yogurt per avocado (optional)*
- *salt and pepper*

Scoop the flesh out of the avocado into a bowl. Add all of the other ingredients and mash together or use a blender for a smoother texture. Season to taste.

Serve in a bowl with a garnish of coriander leaves.

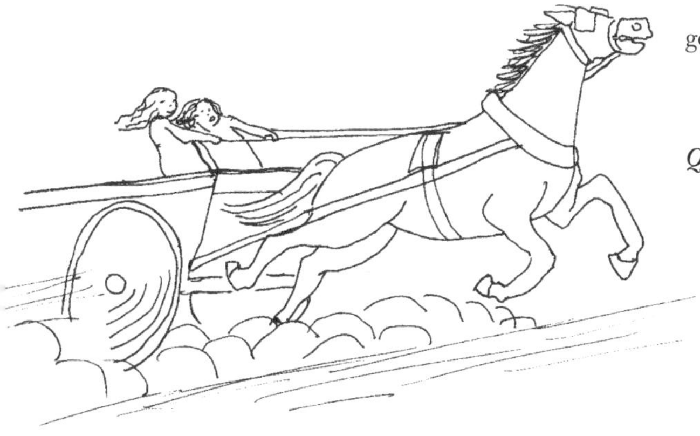

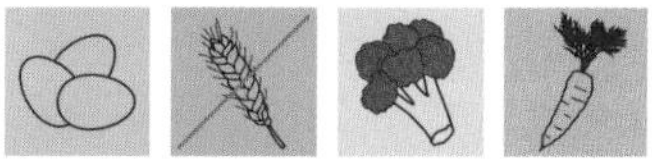

Easy muffins

moderate oven

makes 12

Making puddings for people who can't eat fruit can be difficult. These easy muffins will fill the gap. They also make good birthday and picnic fare.

- *110g (4oz) sifted gluten-free flour*
- *3 tsp gluten-free baking powder*
- *pinch of xanthan gum*
- *60g (2oz) maple syrup*
- *110ml (4fl oz) oil*
- *2 eggs*
- *1 tsp vanilla essence*

Heat the oven to 180°C/ fan160°C/350°F/Gas 4 and grease a 12-hole muffin tin.

Add all the ingredients to a bowl and stir together to make a sloppy mix, then pour into the holes of the muffin tin.

Bake in the oven for 10–15 minutes or until risen and golden brown. Transfer to a wire rack to cool.

Quick, get me out of here, someone is peeling an orange!

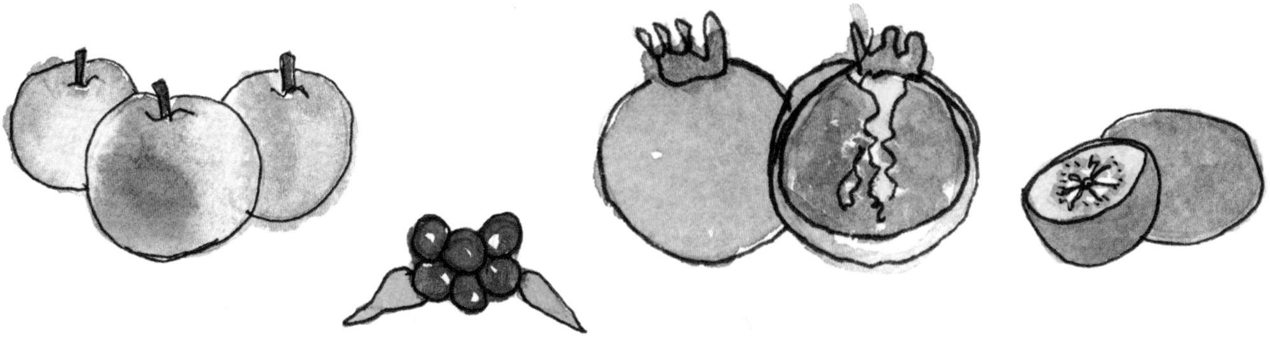

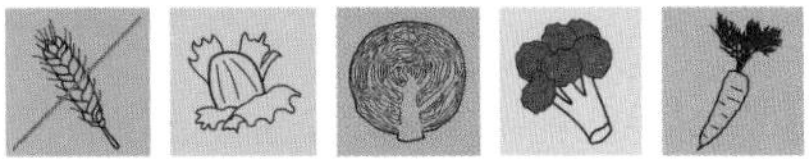

Raw ginger slice

serves 4

A tasty addition to fruit salad for those who can eat fruit or an alternative pudding for those who cannot.

- *125g (4½oz) cashew nuts*
- *125g (4½oz) almonds*
- *125g (4½oz) desiccated coconut*
- *125g (4½oz) pitted dates*
- *1 tsp ground ginger*
- *1 tsp grated fresh root ginger (optional)*
- *2 tsp vanilla paste*
- *1 tsp salt*
- *1 tsp lemon zest (optional)*

In a blender, separately blend the cashews, then the almonds and then the dried coconut until they each reach a flour-like consistency.

Add all the ingredients to the blender and whiz together. If the mix doesn't stick together, add some water a drop at a time until it does.

Line a baking tray (20 x 20cm/8 x 8in) with greaseproof paper and press the mix in, uniformly. Mark the mixture into squares with a sharp knife and transfer to the fridge to firm up before serving with ice-cream.

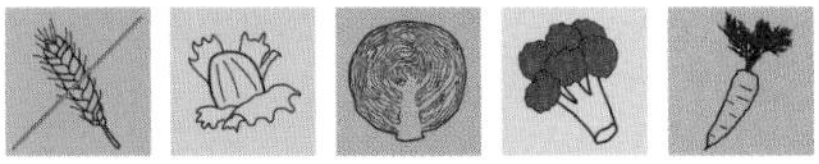

Vegan chocolate cheesecake

freezer

serves 4–6

This is a raw food recipe if you use raw cacao. Replace the honey with agave if you are making this for vegan meal. Enjoy the luxurious taste and creamy texture.

Base

- *350g (12oz) hazelnuts*
- *13 pitted dates*
- *3 tbsp agave syrup (or honey if not for vegans)*
- *2 tsp cocoa powder*

Chocolate layer

- *3 avocados*
- *3 tbsp coconut cream*
- *9 tbsp cocoa powder*
- *3 tbsp agave syrup (or honey if not for vegans)*

Roast the hazelnuts in a dry frying pan or on a tray in a hot oven for 10 minutes until golden brown. Tip onto a plate and allow to cool.

Put all the ingredients into a blender and blend together just until they make a dough. Press the mixture into a 20cm (8in) greaseproof-lined springform cake tin and put in the fridge to chill and set while you make the topping.

Blend all the chocolate layer ingredients together until smooth. Pour onto the chilled base layer and smooth out. Cover with cling film and place in the freezer for 1 hour before serving.

Serve cold on the springform base.

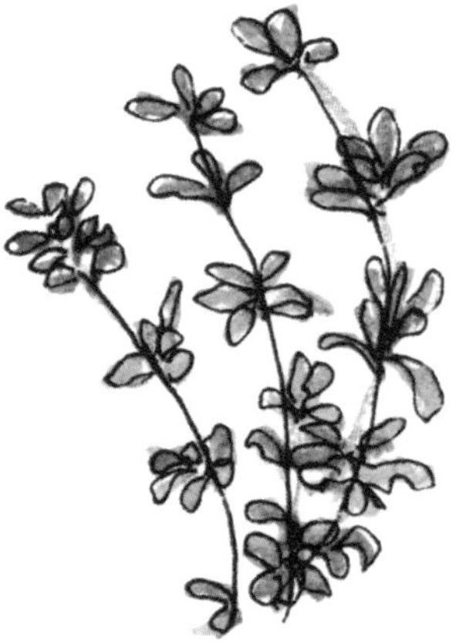

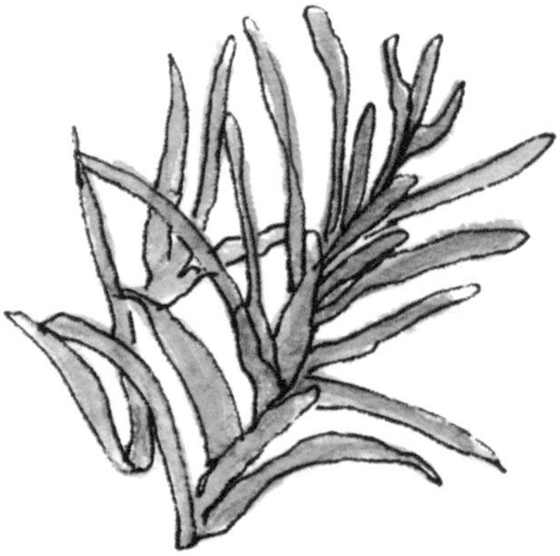

HERBS

The peoples who lived in the British Isles before the arrival of the Romans used few herbs and spices – there was mountain thyme, bog myrtle and wild garlic. The Romans introduced many of the herbs and vegetables that we now cook with, including black mustard, rosemary, thyme, garlic, bay, basil, borage and garden mint.

Herbs give instant flavour, and some are so redolent of certain foods you can trick a person into believing that a meal contains ingredients that are not really there. For instance, you can trick a meat-eater into thinking there really is lamb in that vegetable pie by using lots of onions and rosemary.

Traditionally herbs were part of everyday cooking but, as we became industrialised and separated from the land, we began to use fewer and fewer fresh herbs. Now we are sold packets of dried mixes for tacos, pasta or pizza. But it doesn't have to be like that.

It is worthwhile growing your own herbs even if you have little space or patience to grow anything else. You can buy packets of seeds and compost and sow your own in yogurt pots and keep them on a sunny windowsill – either outside in summer or inside if you don't have access. The plants need to be watered regularly but not more than most houseplants. Some herbs are over in one season (basil, coriander, cress, rocket) and some last year in year out with careful cutting (rosemary, thyme, sage, bay).

There is a great satisfaction in using something that you have nurtured into maturity. In my garden at the moment

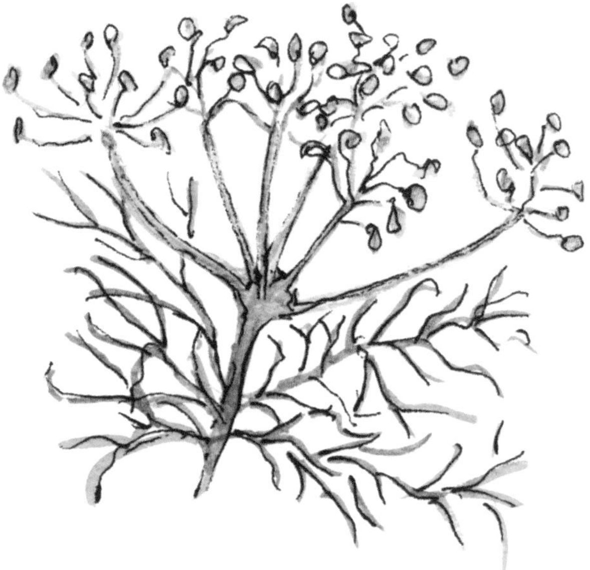

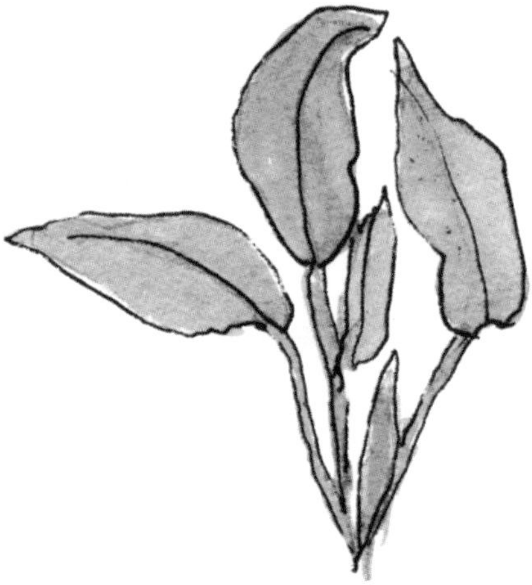

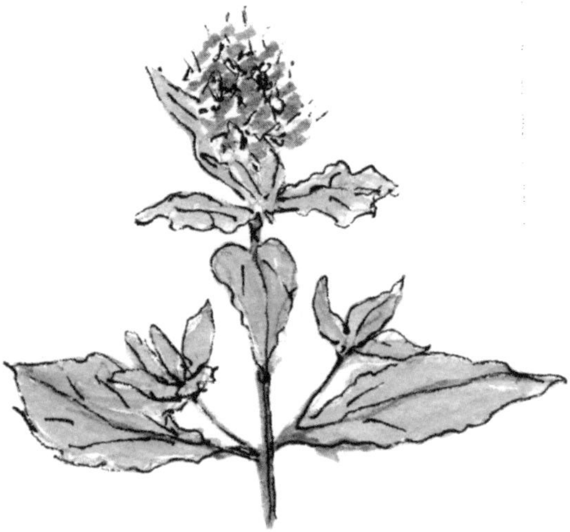

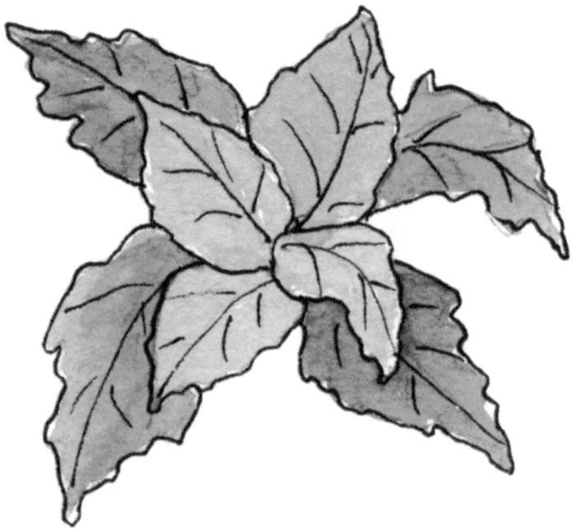

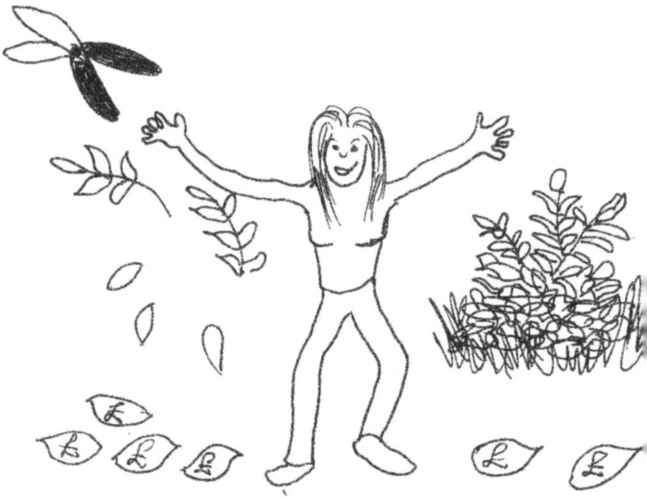

I could be a bay leaf millionaire!

I am growing rosemary, thyme, parsley, sage, marjoram, oregano, basil, cress, bay, nasturtium, mustard, fennel, chives, chervil, four different mints, lovage and rocket – all of which I use in everyday cooking but which come into their own to add extra taste to vegan or vegetarian dishes. I was trimming the bay tree one year and worked out that if I dried and packaged the leaves and managed to sell them all, I would be a bay leaf millionaire!

If you don't have time or space to grow from seed, buy some of the growing herbs from a supermarket and carefully separate the seedlings in several pots to grow on. This works for living salads, too, as lettuces are very forgiving about having their roots disturbed.

Most recipes call for 1 teaspoon of this or that dried herb but in restaurants they use fresh herbs by the handful, so don't be afraid to add more. Keep tasting to make sure you are not overwhelming other flavours, but generally herbs enhance rather than detract from deliciousness.

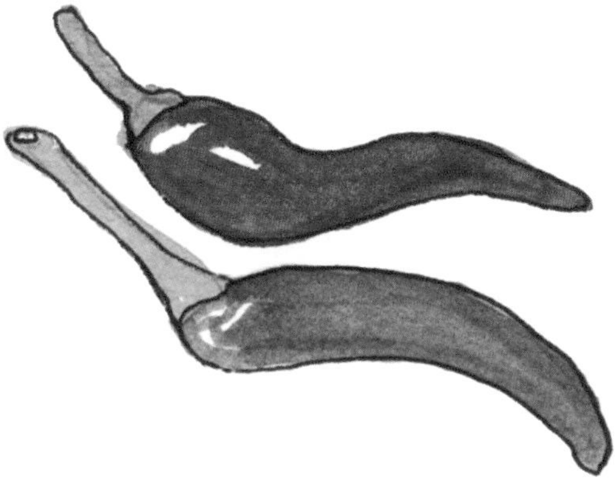

Spices

While the Roman invaders gave us many herbs, it was the Normans who brought spices to our shores. These included cinnamon, saffron, mace, nutmeg, pepper, ginger and sugar. Then the British Raj brought curry spices to the UK: the Hindoostane Coffee House was the first Indian restaurant to open in London, in 1810.

Spices add piquancy and depth of flavour to both savoury and sweet dishes. On my spice shelf are all the separate ingredients for curries, oriental dishes and sweet bakes, but I also have curry powders and pastes because every single spice and every blend gives its own flavour.

The only spices I grow are coriander, fennel, caraway and chilli, because generally spices need more warmth than we get outdoors in the UK. But if you have access to a greenhouse or polytunnel you could try to grow ginger and lemongrass.

RECIPES

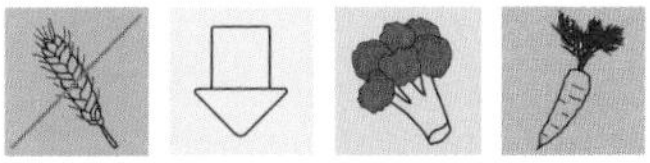

Mild curry powder

There are many mild curry powders for sale; some have fenugreek, some celery powder, some paprika. If you have family or friends with sensitivities, it is best to make your own. This makes a small amount which is best for freshness. For the fullest taste, use fresh packets of spices to make this. Other spices can be added to curries alongside this basic mix.

- *2 tsp ground coriander*
- *3 tsp ground cumin*
- *2 tsp ground turmeric*
- *1 tsp ground fenugreek*
- *3 ground cardamom*
- *1 tsp onion seeds (optional)*
- *¼ tsp chilli powder*

Put all the powders together in a bowl and mix well.

Place in an airtight jar until using in a recipe.

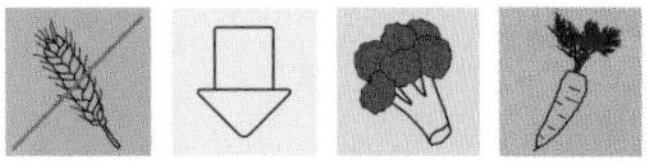

Moroccan spice mix

I've seen Moroccan spice mix with paprika, ginger, black pepper, coriander, cardamon, allspice, mace and nutmeg or with just cumin, cinnamon and mint. By mixing your own you can add any spices you like or take out the ones you don't. Then you get back what you put in!

- *15g each of ground turmeric, chilli, cinnamon, grated nutmeg*
- *30g each of ground black pepper, cumin, ginger*

Put all the powders together in a bowl and mix well.

Place in an airtight jar until using in a recipe.

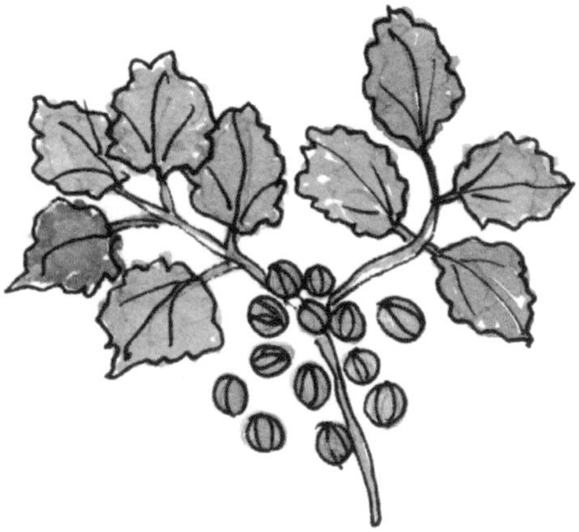

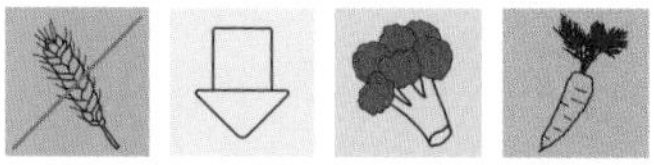

Sweet chilli dipping sauce

serves 4

Versatile and very quick to make, this can change an ordinary stir-fry into a special dish.

- *1 garlic clove, pressed*
- *1 red chilli, deseeded and finely chopped*
- *50g (2oz) caster sugar, honey or maple syrup*
- *3 tbsp white wine vinegar*
- *1 tsp tamari (optional)*
- *100ml (3½fl oz) water*

Place all the ingredients in a small saucepan. Boil rapidly for 8–10 minutes, until the chilli is soft and the sauce is reduced by half. Pour into a small dish and cool before serving.

As an alternative add 1 teaspoon of chopped spring onion and a sprig of coriander before serving.

Serve with rice and noodle dishes.

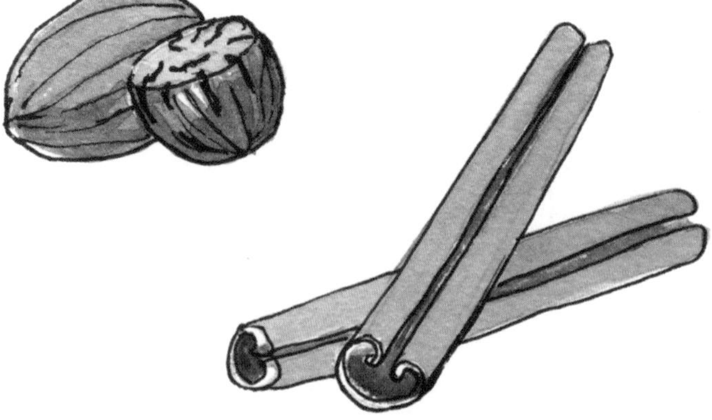

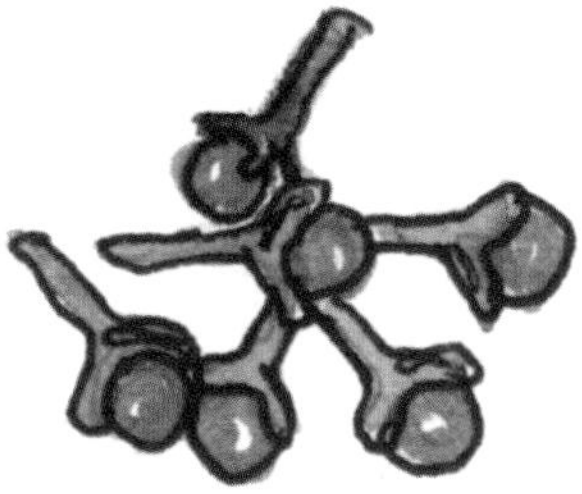

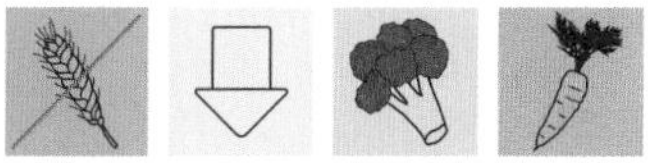

Spicy potatoes

stove top & oven

serves 4

Serve as a side dish with curries. Using the same spices as here, this can make spicy cauliflower or spicy sweet potatoes for those not eating potatoes. Use any leftover to make spicy burgers or as a base for curried vegetable pasties.

- *1 tbsp olive oil, for roasting*
- *1 tsp salt*
- *1 tsp each of chilli powder, fennel seed, onion seed, coriander seed*
- *1 tbsp ground turmeric*
- *3cm (1¼in) piece of fresh root ginger, finely grated*
- *3 garlic cloves, pressed*
- *600g (1lb 5oz) potatoes cut into 2cm (¾in) cubes*

Heat the oven to 180°C/ fan160°C/350°F/Gas 4. In a large roasting tin, mash together the oil, salt, spices, ginger and garlic. Add the potatoes and cover them all over with the mash. Roast for 30 minutes or until golden brown.

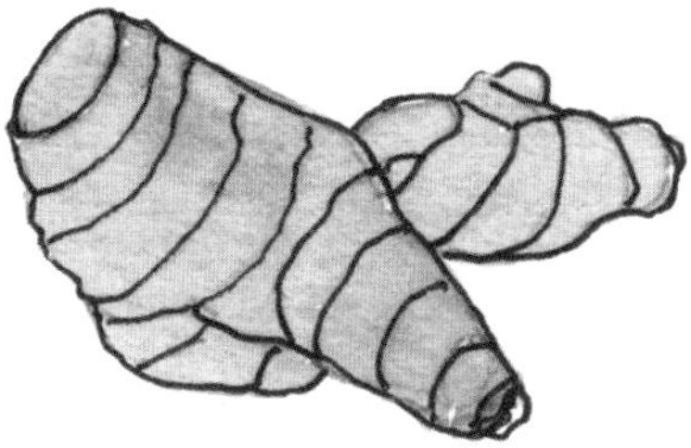

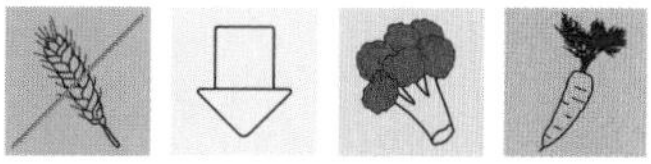

Vegetable curry

stove top

serves 4

If serving this to meat eaters, fry or roast the meat separately and use the curry as a poured over sauce. Once you have made this a few times, experiment with different spice combinations and amounts, especially cumin, turmeric, onion seed and curry leaves

- *1 carrot*
- *1 onion*
- *2 potatoes*
- *3 runner beans or handful of peas or spinach*
- *1 tbsp oil, for frying*
- *1 tbsp mild curry powder*
- *pinch of salt*
- *1 tbsp tomato purée (optional)*
- *1 tbsp chopped coriander (cilantro) leaves*

Cut all the veg into various sized pieces. Carrots can be small, potatoes larger, onions in strips or rings. Place them all in a large pan and simmer for 10 minutes.

In heavy pan fry all the ingredients in the oil together with the curry powder and salt. Add the tomato purée, if using, and fry for 1 minute. Add enough water to make thick sauce and simmer for 30 minutes or until all is cooked.

Adjust the seasoning and add coriander before serving.

SPECIAL DIETS

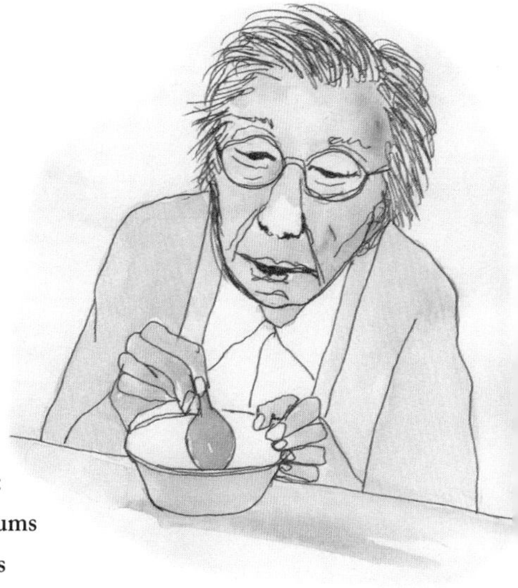

There are as many different diets as there are people and it is only recently that this has come to be respected. If she felt she couldn't eat what was on her plate as a child, my mother was told to 'like it or lump it'. I was told about the starving millions, when I spurned any foods and my children were cajoled or bribed to eat 'just three more mouthfuls, then you can have pudding'.

Recently, I told a doctor friend about *My Family and Other Allergies*, and she said, 'I hope you have included a recipe for those with interstitial cystitis!' I haven't, but I can tell you that many people with IC do not consume coffee, soda, alcohol, fruit juices, hot peppers or spicy foods. Surprisingly, sauerkraut, cranberry juice and yogurt are on the list of most bothersome foods for them.

According to data from YouGov, 43 per cent of UK adults felt confident that they would be able to cook ten or more meals from memory, without consulting a recipe book. Older people felt more able than younger. This implies that we have a repertoire which we can more or less stick to, week by week. Whether our guests or family members are choosing to eliminate certain foods for religious, ethnicity, ethical, psychological or health reasons, we may have to go out of our comfort zone and use unfamiliar ingredients to cook for them. Dog-earing the most useful chapters here will provide a great aid to memory and can spark off new inspiration too.

This section covers:

- **Breastfeeding mums**
- **Low-calorie diets**
- **Diabetes and sugar**
- **Gluten intolerance**
- **FODMAP**
- **GAPS diet**
- **The gut biome and IBD (inflammatory bowel disease)**
- **Ethical eating**
- **Vegetarians**
- **Vegans**

A traditional cookbook with its specific ingredients can limit our thinking and self-reliance. These recipes seek to encourage you towards experimentation, a prerequisite to being a good cook, if not a creative genius in your own kitchen. The recipes in this section may mention particular ingredients that the person you are cooking for cannot eat. Sometimes a variation is given in the recipe, but you can often use a substitute anyway. For instance, maple syrup can stand in for honey if your guests are vegan, as in Baked Apples (diabetes and sugar). Soya, almond or oat milk can be substituted for milk in Curried Vegetable Patties (ethical eaters).

As we come to recognise that the food we eat, and how we eat it, influences our physical health and psychological wellbeing, people are more willing to accommodate special diets. And it helps to understand why people choose their various diets, whether they are concerned with their own gut health and wellbeing, or the health and welfare of the planet. It certainly makes for excellent mealtime conversation!

BREASTFEEDING MUMS

Let's hear it for breastfeeding mums. In pregnancy they were sick from certain foods, had heartburn from others and now their little one can't tolerate onions and garlic – or it could be lactose or gluten or cabbages or nuts? Do all babies get wind? What is the difference between wind and colic? Whatever is going on, if you are cooking for someone who is breastfeeding, it is best to assume the worst and go for a meal with none of the above.

A baby's gut is still in development for the first six months or so of their life. During this time, there are spaces between the cells of the gut where certain products from their mother's milk, such as antibodies, can leak through, unfiltered, into the baby's bloodstream. Until the gut has matured, some molecules of other things can get through. Some large molecules can be passed wholesale from the mother's milk into the baby's immature gut, causing it to remain difficult to digest and consequently a cause for pain or vomiting – or a mix of all of these.

The initial stage of gut colonisation during and after birth plays an important part in shaping the future health of an infant. Breastfed infants have a different microbial signature to formula-fed infants and this could explain some of the immune-enhancing protection that breastfeeding offers. Breast milk contains a diverse population of bacteria, but it is only recently beginning to be understood just how phenomenal a mother's milk is. It is a liquid food which changes according to the baby's needs via feedback from their saliva to have more or less fat, sugars or antibodies at different times.

A study* involving over a hundred breastfeeding mother-infant pairs measured the bacterial communities growing in the gut of the infant in the first few months after birth.

Your baby is what you eat.

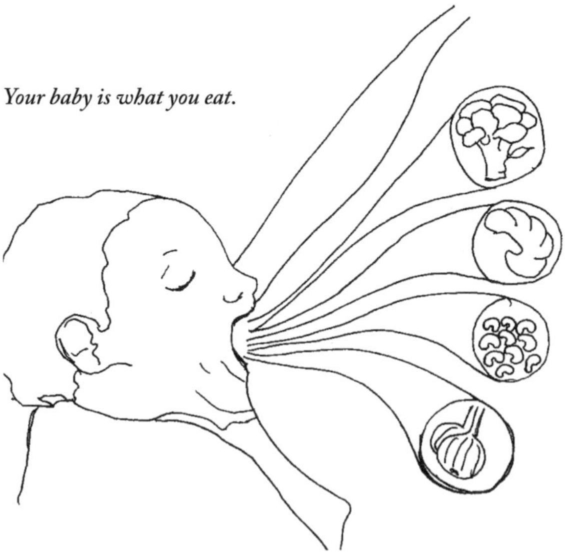

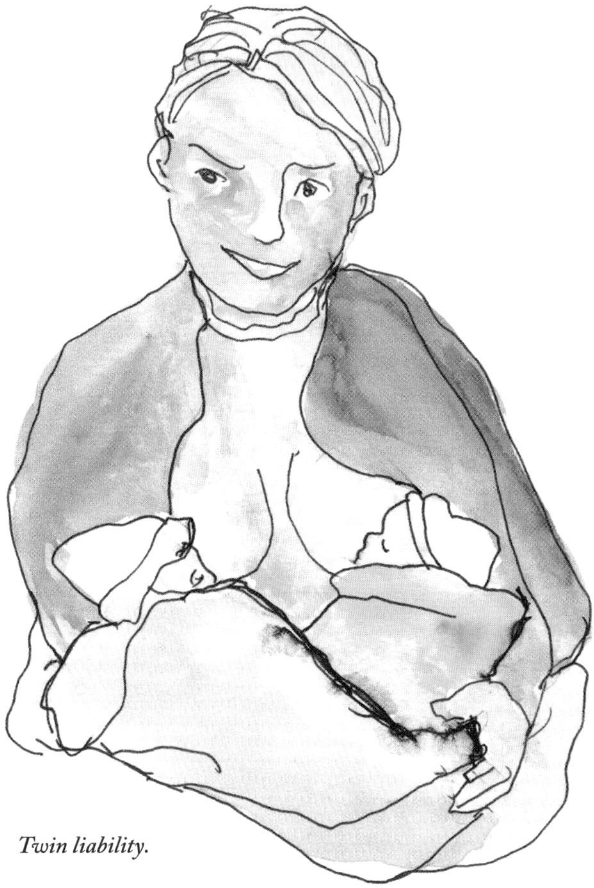

Twin liability.

In the breastfed infants, 28 per cent of the gut bacteria were found to originate from breast milk. A further 10 per cent of bacteria actually came from the skin around the mother's nipple. Adding up to almost 40 per cent, breastfeeding is clearly an important source of bacteria for an infant.

Bacterial diversity is an indicator for a healthy microbiome. Infants who are breastfed have been found to have a more diverse microbiome and this increases with the amount of milk they receive each day – even in the weaning period when solids are being introduced.

Most mothers of breastfed babies have to give up one or two foods until the baby is weaned, and a conscientious breastfeeding mum can track her baby's digestive health and withdraw foods which give pain, giving herself a chance of quieter evenings and nights at the same time as providing the best growing food that her baby could have.

**JAMA Pediatrics, 8 May 2017*

Stella

Stella has two older boys who were both breastfed. One eats almost everything he is served and the other will eat very little of anything (see his story in Fussy Eaters, page 43). She also has twins, one of whom will eat almost anything she is presented with, while the other is fussy.

When Stella started breastfeeding the twins, it was quickly apparent that while Mary couldn't tolerate bovine dairy, Rosie couldn't tolerate wheat. So, after several nights holding one or other colicky baby, Stella gave up milk and wheat. She still eats rye bread and uses sheep's and goat's cheese and milk substitutes and is still breastfeeding. Though the twins have almost self-weaned, Stella continues to limit wheat and dairy until she stops breastfeeding because they seem better without them.

Eventually the nights have become quieter but the days certainly noisier.

The foods that I know that are most likely to cause problems include many acid fruits, such as oranges; dairy products, especially from cows; onions and garlic; gluten-rich cereals, the cabbage family; eggs; and chocolate.

Not all foods cause problems for all babies; some babies have more difficulty and some have none.

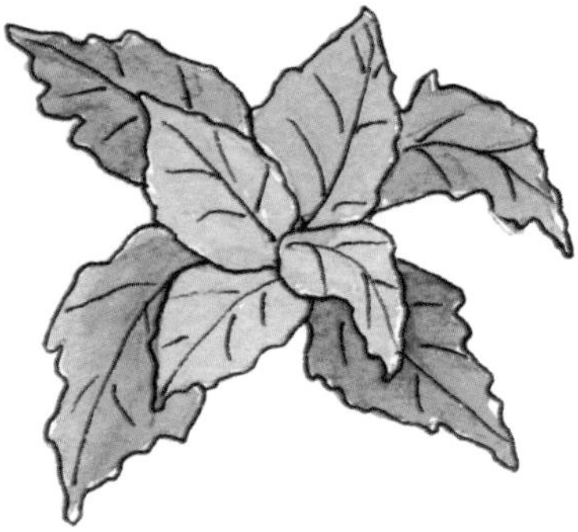

Bought bread

freezer

Using shop-bought sliced bread or whole loaf: choose bread that has the least additives and preservatives. Separate the slices or cut the whole loaf into slices. Place them on a tray and freeze. Once frozen, put the slices into freezer bags and remove single slices whenever they are needed.

You can use the slices as pizza bases or open sandwiches or grate them into crumbs to be a topping for savoury or sweet dishes.

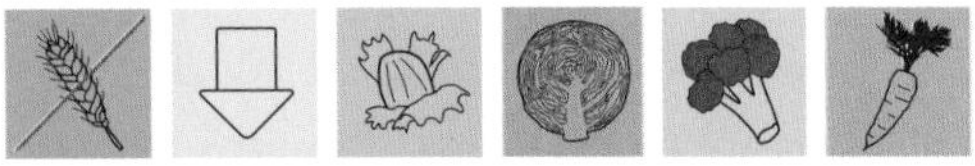

Carrot & coriander salad

per person

- *½ medium carrot, finely or roughly grated, to taste*
- *1 tsp lemon juice or cider vinegar (optional)*
- *1 tbsp toasted sesame seeds (optional)*
- *1 tbsp freshly chopped coriander (cilantro)*
- *1 tsp coriander seeds, crushed*
- *salt and pepper*

Mix together all the ingredients in a bowl and adjust the flavours to taste.

Fresh carrots will be juicier than old ones, so add a little water if it seems dry.

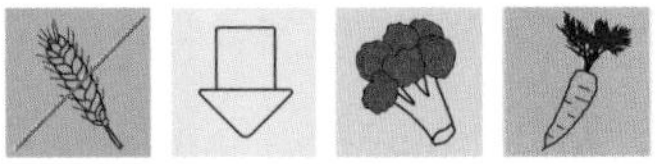

Quinoa salad

stove top

Quinoa is unique in having all the essential amino acids that the body needs and is naturally gluten free.

- *110g (4oz) quinoa*
- *1 tsp finely chopped rosemary*
- *1 tsp finely chopped thyme*
- *1 courgette (zucchini), finely sliced*
- *1 red onion, finely sliced*
- *1 red pepper, chopped (optional)*
- *110g (4oz) rocket (arugula) leaves*
- *3 tbsp chopped basil*
- *4 lemon wedges and a handful of toasted pine nuts (optional)*

Rinse and drain the quinoa, bring to the boil and simmer with the rosemary and thyme for 10 minutes until done. Then drain in a sieve and rinse with cold water.

Fry the courgette and onion and pepper (if using) in a frying pan until just cooked.

In a salad bowl, mix the quinoa with the vegetables and scatter with the rocket and basil.

Serve cold with lemon wedges and pine nuts for extra crunch, if you like.

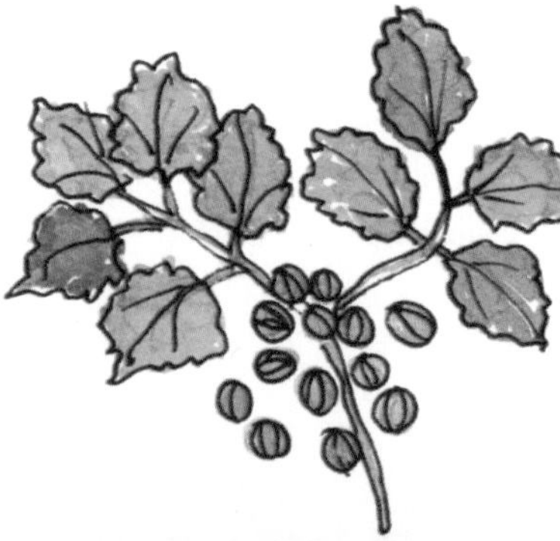

Spinach with dill

stove top

- *350g (12oz) washed, chopped spinach (if using chard remove stalks)*
- *2 tbsp finely chopped dill*
- *1 tsp pine nuts (optional)*
- *salt and pepper*

Place the spinach with the water left on the leaves after washing in a pan. Set over a low heat, put the lid on and steam for 5–10 minutes.

Once cooked, add the chopped dill and pine nuts, if using, and season to taste.

Burger 1 (portobello mushroom)

stove top

- *1 or 2 portobello mushrooms per person*
- *1 garlic clove, finely chopped*
- *oil, for frying*
- *½ onion, sliced into rings*
- *1 beef tomato, sliced*
- *bun sliced in half, or large lettuce leaves, to serve*
- *your preferred sauces (ketchup and mayo type)*
- *salt and pepper*

Remove the stalks from the mushrooms and fry them in garlic and oil on both sides until crispy and brown. In the same pan, if possible at the same time, fry the onion rings until soft. Add the stalks and any trimmings to the onions as you fry.

In a different frying pan, dry fry the tomato slices until brown on the outside.

Layer all the ingredients between two halves of the bun or rolled lettuce leaves, season and finish with your sauce of choice.

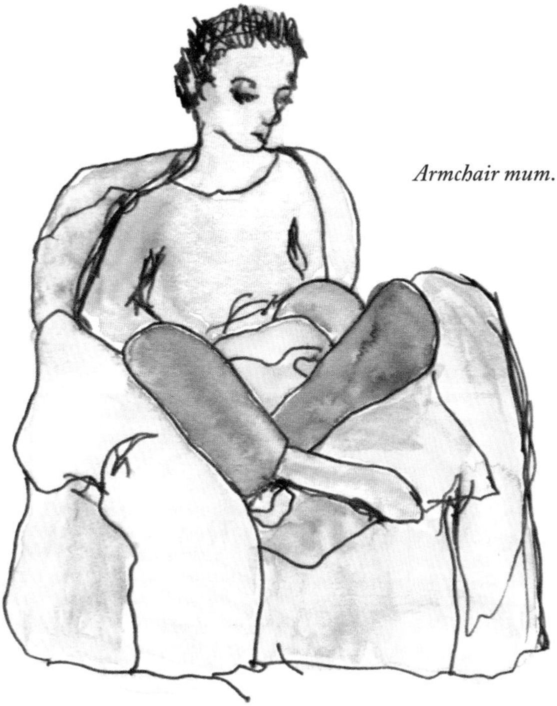

Armchair mum.

BBQ peaches

barbeque / stove top

- *1 peach per person, firm but ripe, stoned and quartered*
- *1 tbsp rose water / orange water*
- *cashew nut cream, to serve*

Place the peach wedges on the grill of the barbecue or on a hot griddle pan, brush with rose or orange water and cook for 4–5 minutes. Repeat on the other juicy side.

Serve hot with cashew nut cream (see page 32).

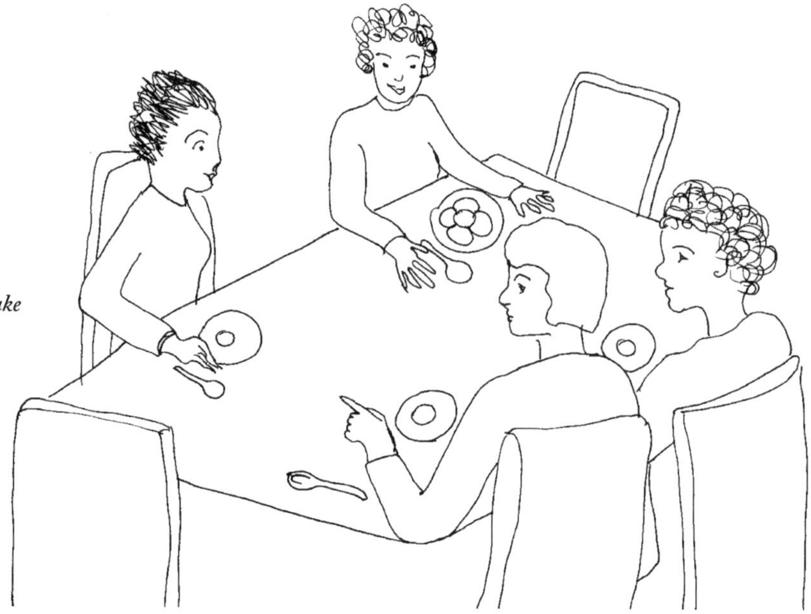

Your plate's empty!

'I know… that cream cake at brunch gave me my 550 calories for today.'

LOW-CALORIE DIETS

People choose a low-calorie diet for many reasons. Some are recommended to do so by their GPs, who then monitor their progress, while some get support from organisations such as WW UK (formerly Weight Watchers UK).

I choose to be on a low-calorie diet regularly and today I am fasting. That means I will not eat anything until around 7pm tonight. It is now almost 3pm and I am struggling to keep up a positive attitude. Sometimes it is not difficult, but today it is. Sometimes it helps to tell myself, 'I can do this, this is a good thing and I am okay with it'. But today it isn't helping and the growling in my belly is growing deeper and louder.

I started fasting about seven years ago and, ever since, every Sunday and Monday I try to cut my calorific intake by just under two-thirds of the recommended intake for a woman of my age. So that means I can eat around 550 calories on these days.

For the first year I would split that between three meals like this:

- **Breakfast** – a hard-boiled egg or very small bowl of porridge made with water.
- **Lunch** – a small, boiled potato and a lot of lettuce drizzled with balsamic vinegar.
- **Supper** – a small bowl of brown rice with steamed vegetables.

Then I tried fasting for the whole day and eating a bigger supper. This suits me fine as I then can sleep through the night without being hungry. For me, a 550-calorie meal seems almost like a normal meal if there is no oil in the dressing and no fried food. And supposedly the longer you can fast between meals the better it is for you – up to a point, of course.

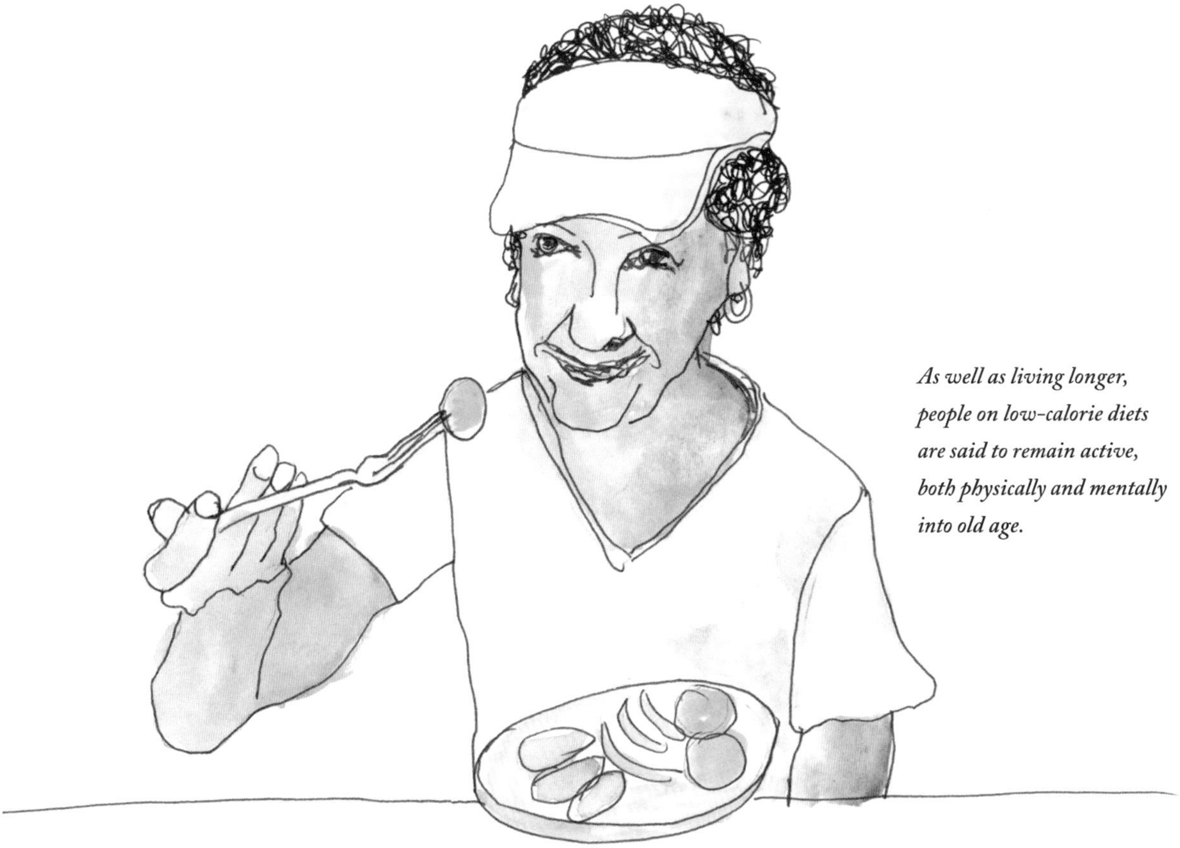

As well as living longer, people on low-calorie diets are said to remain active, both physically and mentally into old age.

The 5:2 fasting diet was popularised by Michael Mosley in the UK in 2012 after it was featured on the BBC2 Horizon documentary Eat, Fast and Live Longer. I saw this programme and it somehow made enough sense for me to try it out, and it has suited me ever since.

Humans have an evolutionary bias towards feasting and fasting from way back when we were hunter-gatherers. The idea behind intermittent fasting is that the cells of our body have a mechanism of growth and repair. When we feast, we switch to growth, and when we fast, we switch to repair. Today we hardly ever fast, so we are permanently aligned towards growth, which means that cells do not get a chance to repair themselves. Then the damage to cells in our various organs may manifest as inflammatory diseases and cancers.

Intermittent fasting does help control my weight, but more than that I feel better when I have been fasting. That is, I feel more alert and alive, generally – though on fast days please do not take offence if I am a little intense!

There are other time-restricted diets, such as the 16:8 – which is thought to resemble the circadian rhythm. People on this diet eat an evening meal and then wait 16 hours before breaking their fast the next day. Imagine missing breakfast and eating a late lunch. The idea is to eat a healthy diet during the eating period and drink calorie-free beverages like water or unsweetened teas and coffee. The 16:8 diet is said to support weight loss and improve blood sugar, brain function and longevity.

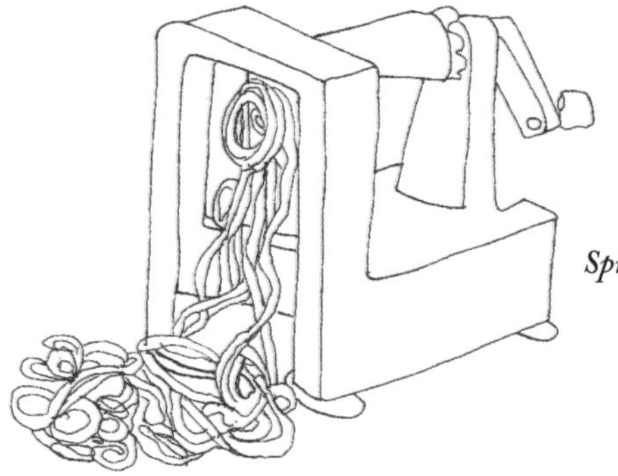

Spiralizer

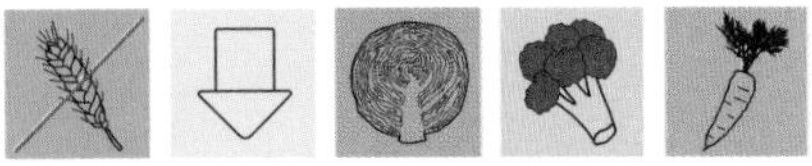

Spiralised veggies

These can be eaten raw as salads or steamed as 'pasta'. Use carrot, beetroot or courgette (zucchini) and use one per person. Serve raw and cold with a mayo-type sauce or steam for 5 minutes and serve hot with a pasta sauce of choice.

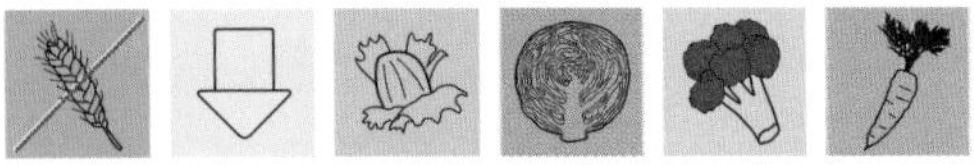

Lizzie's pesto sauce

serves 4

Packed with fresh, nutritious herbs, it feels like you have eaten a full meal after a small amount of this on salads. Delicious as a cold sauce on spiralised vegetables.

- *50g (2oz) cashew nuts*
- *3 big sorrel leaves, chopped*
- *2 small kale leaves, chopped*
- *juice of 1 lemon*
- *1 garlic clove, chopped (optional)*
- *olive oil (optional)*
- *2 tomatoes, finely chopped*
- *salt and pepper*

Blend all the ingredients together in a blender – except the tomatoes. Add a little water or olive oil if the pesto is too stiff.

Add the finely chopped tomatoes just before serving.

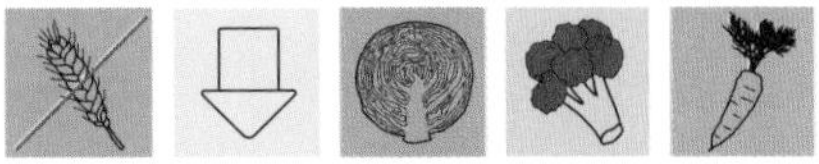

Raw tomato relish

serves 4

A low-calorie alternative to salad dressing with oil or to sweet chutney, this has a lot of flavour.

As an alternative, add 1 tablespoon of diced cucumber and 1 tablespoon of chopped basil with 1 tablespoon of tamari and 1 tablespoon of water.

- *1 large tomato, diced*
- *1 onion, finely chopped*
- *1 garlic clove, finely chopped (optional)*
- *1 sprig of coriander (cilantro) or basil, chopped*
- *1 tbsp cider vinegar*

Combine all the ingredients in a shallow bowl.

Serve as a side dish with rice dishes or baked potatoes.

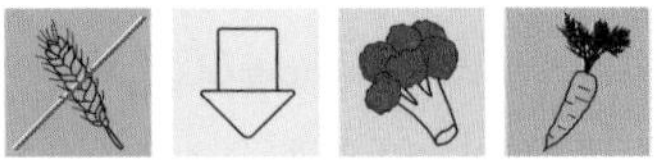

Steamed vegetables

stove top

serves 4

Delicious for a post-fast meal or a low-calorie day.

- *1kg (2¼lb) mix of any roughly chopped carrots, onion, swede, turnip, carrot*

Steam all the vegetables together for around 10 minutes or until cooked but still crunchy.

Serve with rice and a tomato sauce or alongside a pie.

Meg's vegetable loaf

oven

serves 4–6

When it is sliced, the colours of the layers and the aroma of the vegetables make this a luxury low-calorie dish fit for a wedding or Christmas feast. You could add goat's cheese to the spinach layer for a vegetarian version.

- *2 medium onions, finely chopped*
- *200g chopped spinach*
- *½ tsp grated nutmeg*
- *250g (8oz) beetroot, boiled, then peeled and cut into 5mm slices*
- *250g (8oz) butternut squash, roasted and cut into 5mm slices*
- *3 bay leaves*
- *salt and pepper*

Heat the oven to 180°C/ fan160°C/350°F/Gas 4.

Fry the onions until soft and add the spinach, fry a little longer then add the nutmeg and seasoning.

Line a bread tin with greased silver foil, then cover the base with the beetroot slices in one layer. Add a layer of spinach mix followed by a layer of squash. Repeat until the tin is full. Place the bay leaves on the top. Fold the foil over the top and press down gently to compress the loaf.

Bake in the oven for 1 hour.

Remove the top layer of foil and turn the loaf upside down to release it from the tin. Unpeel the rest of the foil and lift the loaf onto a plate. Slice carefully with a sharp knife to serve.

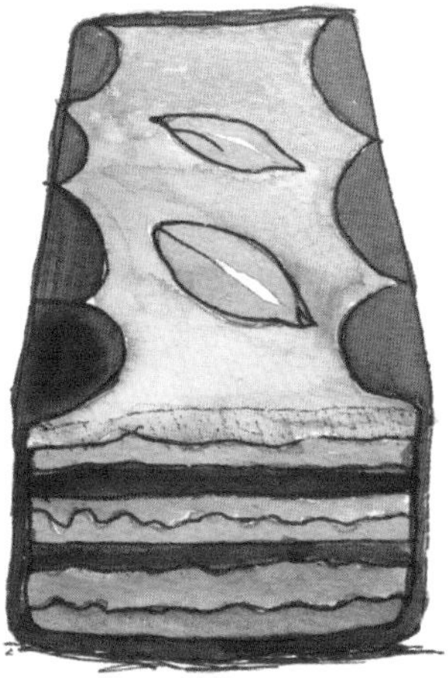

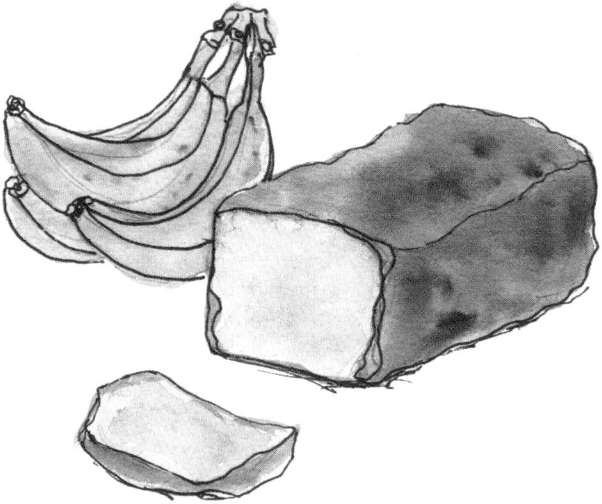

Banana cake – no sugar, no eggs

oven

serves 4-6

This is true luxury and because it has no sugar or eggs a small slice will not upset anyone's low-calorie diet (too much)!

- *80g (3oz) wholewheat or gluten-free plain flour*
- *125g (4½oz) gluten-free self-raising flour*
- *4 tsp baking powder*
- *1 tsp salt*
- *1 tsp grated nutmeg*
- *1 small tsp xanthan gum*
- *225g (8oz) pitted dates, chopped and whizzed up*
- *4 squishy bananas*
- *1 slosh of water or milk substitute*
- *100g (4oz) coconut oil*

Heat the oven to 170°C/ fan150°C/325°F/Gas 3.

Sift all the dry ingredients together into a mixing bowl. Add all the other ingredients and beat everything together until well combined.

Pour into a greaseproof paper-lined loaf tin. Bake at the centre of the oven for about 1 hour or until golden brown and a skewer inserted in the middle comes out clean.

Remove from the tin and cool on a wire rack.

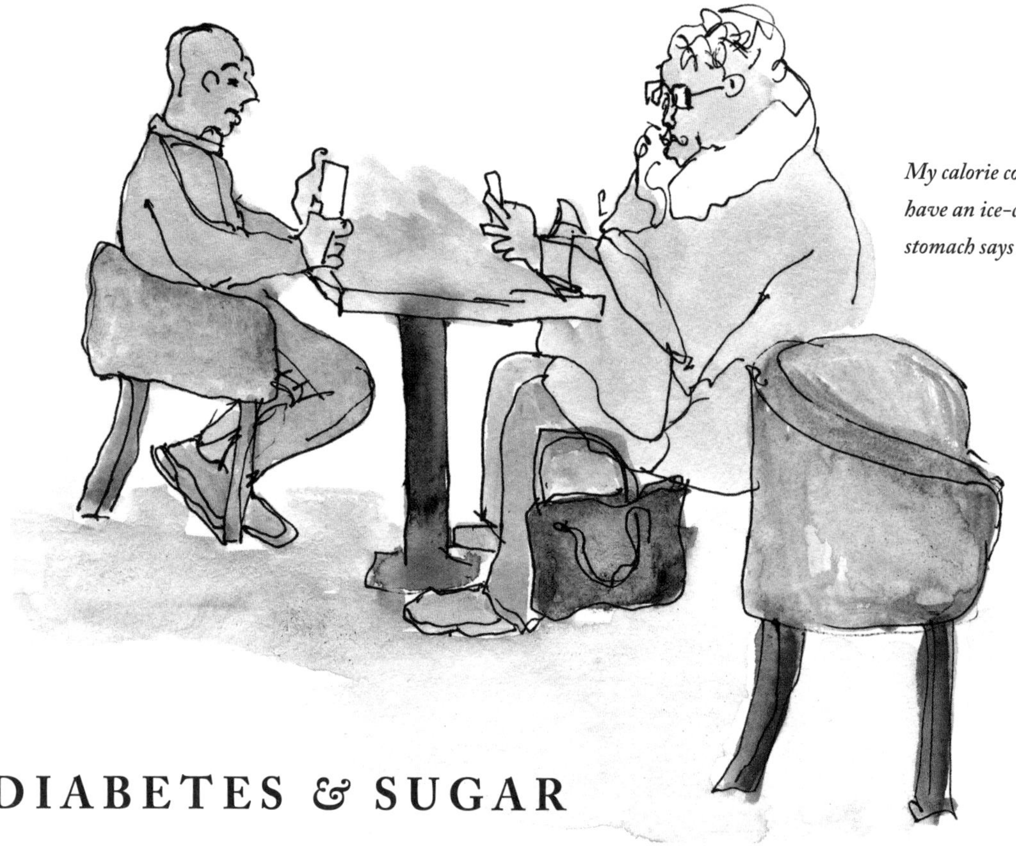

My calorie counter says I can have an ice-cream but my stomach says I can have two.

DIABETES & SUGAR

People with diabetes have blood glucose levels that are too high on occasion. Diabetes is caused by a disfunction of insulin levels made by the pancreas. Insulin causes the liver to convert glucose (a simple sugar) to glycogen (a fat) for storage, thus removing it from the blood.

Having too much blood glucose can lead to the following symptoms: increased thirst, frequent urination, hunger, fatigue, blurred vision, slow wound healing and yeast infections – such as thrush or athlete's foot.

Diabetic diagnoses will be one of two types:

• Diabetes type 1 is a genetic, autoimmune disease where the immune system attacks and destroys cells in the pancreas, thereby rendering it less able to produce insulin. Type 1 is not a condition that develops over time, so most children who are diagnosed with diabetes have type 1. People with type 1 learn to control their diet and avoid foods that create spikes in their blood glucose levels. They also monitor their blood sugar levels and inject themselves with insulin, if need be.

• Diabetes type 2 is a metabolic disorder and happens when a person's body becomes resistant to insulin. This is not genetic or congenital. It is said that nine in every 10 people with diabetes have type 2. Almost 200,000 people a year are diagnosed with type 2 diabetes in England and Wales. Type 2 is linked to obesity and excessive sugar and fat intake. There is so much glucose in the blood and so much fat in and around the liver that it can no longer function properly, so it becomes resistant to insulin.

Recent studies challenge the perception that type 2 diabetes needs to be a lifelong condition for everyone diagnosed with it, and evidence suggests that in obese people weight loss in particular can lead to diabetes remission. Remission happens when blood glucose levels are below the diabetic range, but this doesn't mean that diabetes has gone for good. It's really important for people in remission to get regular healthcare checks, so any complications can be monitored and any signs of type 2 diabetes coming back can be caught early.

Both types of diabetes can be helped by losing weight, reducing sugar and fat intake and taking more exercise.

Mari

It was the Christmas market and two-year-old Mari attracted lots of attention from stallholders and shoppers alike. She was walking around eating a raw Brussels sprout on a stick. Mari cannot tolerate sugar or chocolate or many fats or flours, so her clever mother had given her a sprout as a special treat. This resulted in a happy child and some astounded adults.

Sugar

Strong evidence now shows that eating too much added sugar is a major contributor to diseases such as diabetes, heart disease and liver malfunction. Added sugar is found in around three-quarters of all manufactured foods, including many that are savoury or marked as healthy.

A 2003 World Health Organization (WHO) technical report provided evidence that the high intake of sugary drinks (including fruit juices) increased the risk of obesity by adding to overall calorie intake. Though by itself sugar does not cause obesity, when over consumed it is a leading component of unhealthy diets leading to diabetes. Sugar intake is greater when combined with fats. Non-alcoholic liver disease, which can lead to cirrhosis, is now thought to be present in about a third of all American adults.

Annie

Annie was on a strict diet that involved very few, if any, carbohydrates or vegetables, a lot of butter and a lot of meat protein. This was to heal her leaky gut. However, it turned out that Annie didn't have a leaky gut, as she had thought, but a very irritated one from all the sugar she had been eating. Once she stopped eating sugar, her gut health improved dramatically. Her complexion became clear and her energetic lust for life returned.

Another cake?

No thanks, I eat with my hypothalamus and that tells me I'm full.

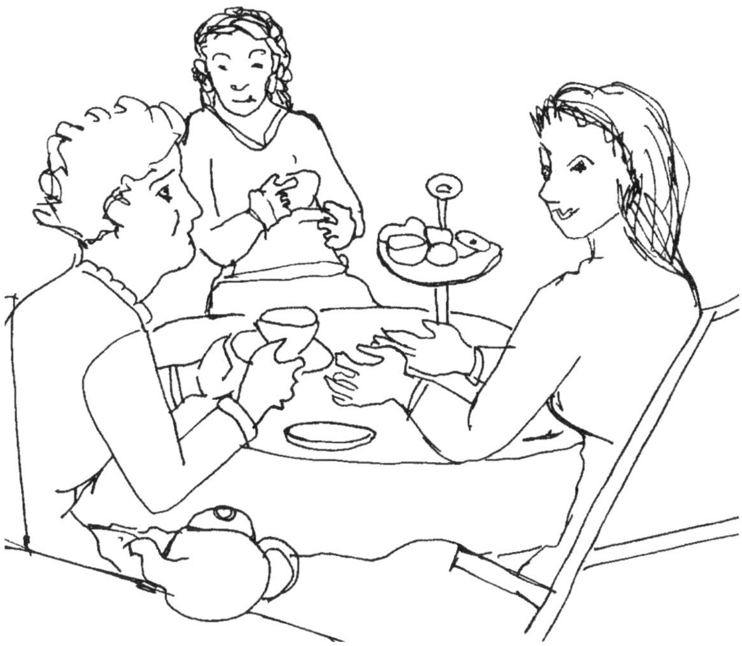

The average person consumes around 500g (1lb 2oz) of sugar a week – more in developed nations and less in developing ones. The WHO recommends a reduction in this level of sugar intake of at least 10 per cent.

A so-called sugar tax was introduced in the UK in 2017 and led to a fall of just under 30 per cent in the amount of sugar in soft drinks. However, it appears that some food producers have increased the amount of sugar in sweets and confectionery and in fact overall sugar consumption rose by 2018.

Elizabeth & Cleopatra

Queen Elizabeth I had blackened, peg-like teeth. Cleopatra's teeth were rotten and Washington had wooden teeth. However the teeth of the peasants and serfs of the Middle Ages and the teeth of Neanderthals were healthy and so were their gums. It appears that poor people who lived close to nature and who had no access to sugar had little or no tooth decay.

A sweet tooth is a fairly modern phenomenon among the world's population, and no longer just an affliction of the rich.

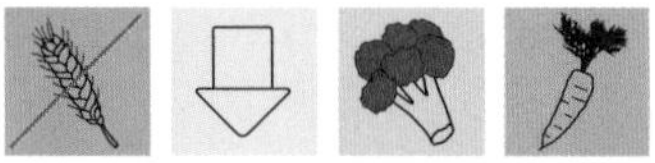

Quick baked beans

stove top

serves 4

Branded baked beans may have between 3–4 teaspoons of sugar per can. This hidden source represents at least 10% of the normal daily intake of sugar.

- *1 tsp minced garlic (optional)*
- *1 tbsp finely chopped onion (optional)*
- *1–2 tsp frying oil*
- *340g (12oz) cooked or tinned flageolet beans*
- *1 tsp dried celery leaf or 1tsp vegan bouillon*
- *2 tbsp tomato purée or chopped tinned tomatoes*
- *salt and pepper*

Sauté the garlic and onion in the oil in a large saucepan until soft. Add the beans and celery leaf or bouillon and tomato purée, stirring well.

Cook for 2 minutes and add enough water to make a thick sauce, then continue cooking for 5 more minutes, season to taste and serve hot.

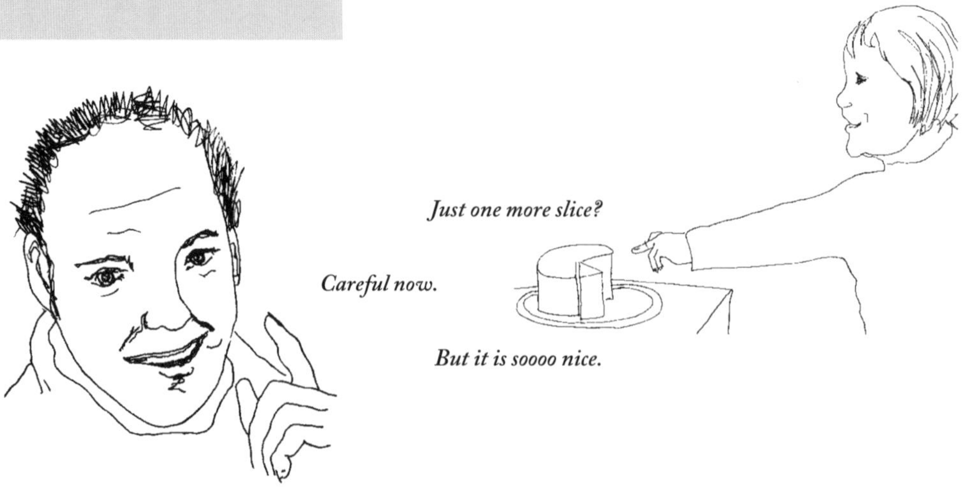

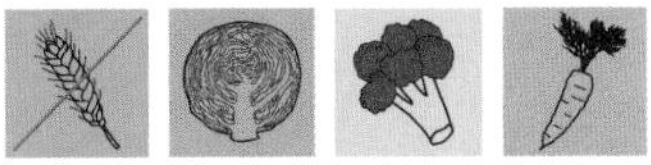

No-vinegar ketchup

stove top

There are 4 grams of sugar in a tablespoon of some branded ketchups. While vinegar is said to benefit people with diabetes by lowering their blood sugars, it is best to take it by itself BEFORE a meal not during.

- *4 tbsp tomato purée*
- *3 tbsp water*
- *1 tbsp sunflower or olive oil*
- *1 garlic clove, pressed*
- *1 tsp date or agave syrup*
- *salt and pepper*

Whiz all the ingredients and seasoning together in a blender until smooth. Add the syrup to taste and transfer to a sterilised bottle or jar with a lid.

This ketchup will keep in the fridge for several days.

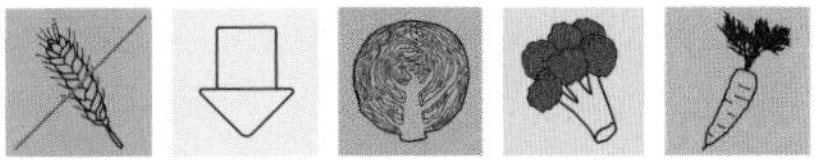

Salted lemons

Almost calorie free but packed with long-lasting flavour.

- *4 lemons*
- *4–5 tbsp salt*

Cut the lemons almost through, lengthways, into 4 or 6 wedges. Transfer to a plate, stand upright and stuff the insides of the lemons with salt. Pack the lemons into mason jars, seal and leave overnight.

Add enough water to top up the juice until it just covers the lemons, then seal again and leave for a month.

Remove and drain the wedges as needed, then slice and dice them and add to tagines, salads and rice dishes.

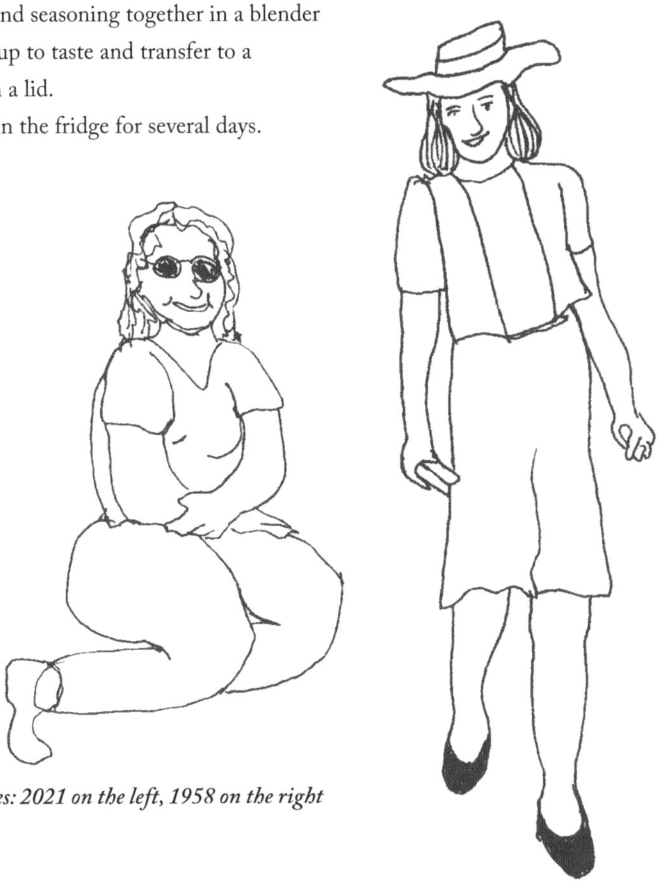

Body shapes: 2021 on the left, 1958 on the right

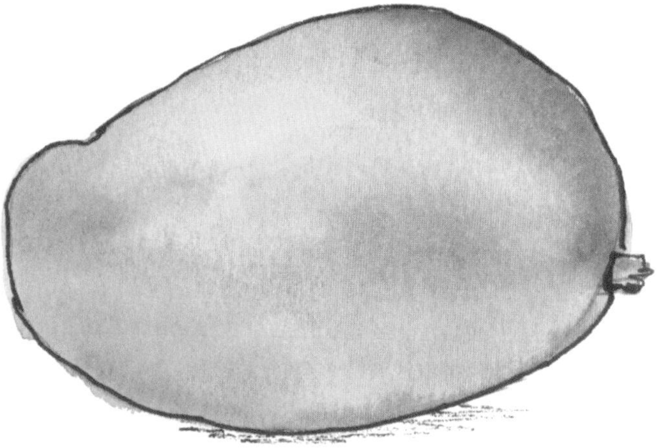

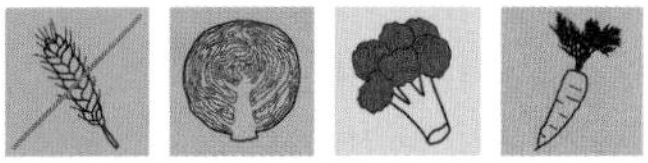

Mango salsa

serves 4

A fresh, super tasty alternative to sugar-loaded chutneys. Serve as a side dish with rice dishes and curries.

- *1 mango, peeled, stoned and flesh chopped into small pieces*
- *½ red onion, finely chopped*
- *2 tbsp chopped coriander (cilantro) leaves*
- *1 garlic clove, finely chopped (optional)*
- *1 finely chopped red chilli (optional)*
- *½ tbsp olive or sunflower oil*
- *½ tbsp lemon or lime juice or cider vinegar*
- *salt and pepper*

Mix all the ingredients together in a bowl except the oil and citrus juice.

Combine the oil and lemon juice or vinegar in a small jug and pour over the salsa. Serve at once.

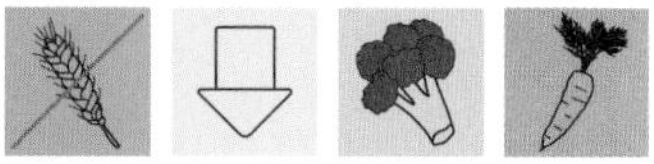

Savoury muffins

moderate oven

serves 4

Hidden sugar in savoury products is of major concern to anyone who is careful with their calorie or sugar intake. Just one cheese and black pepper muffin, from a major supermarket, has a whopping 191 calories and includes among other ingredients: wheat flour, mature cheddar cheese, wheat gluten, cheese powder, yeast, soya flour, salt, sugar and palm oil. Instead of chives, try freshly chopped herbs such as rosemary and thyme.

- *50g (2oz) arrowroot*
- *110g (4oz) rice flour*
- *1 tsp psyllium husk (optional)*
- *4 tsp baking powder*
- *1 tsp xanthan gum*
- *100ml (3½fl oz) cooking oil*
- *2 eggs, beaten*
- *4–6 tbsp soya or rice milk, or enough to make sloppy mix*
- *1 tsp poppy seeds (optional)*
- *1 tsp chopped chives*

Heat the oven to 180°C/ fan160°C/350°F/Gas 4 and grease the holes of a 9-hole muffin tin.

Put everything in a large mixing bowl and stir together to make a sloppy mix, then spoon into the muffin tin. Transfer to the oven and bake for about 10–15 minutes or until risen and golden brown.

Serve with soup.

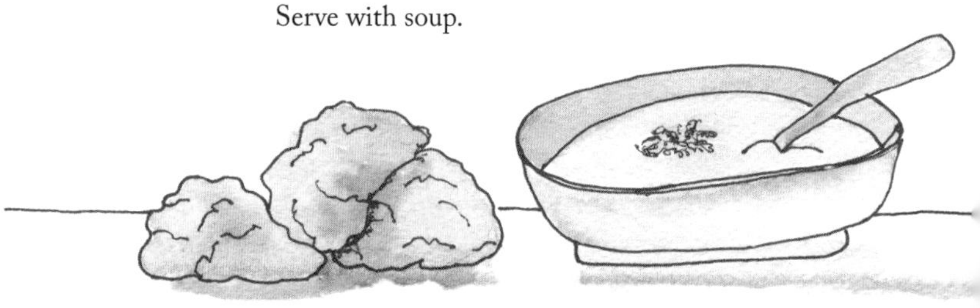

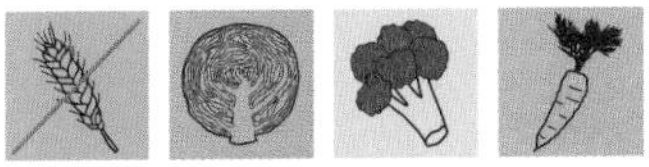

Salad dressing

Commercial dressings are loaded with sugar, salt and saturated fats. Alternatives are expensive and the real thing is ridiculously easy to make.

- *50ml (2fl oz) olive oil*
- *50ml (2fl oz) cider vinegar, lemon juice or balsamic vinegar, or a mix*
- *1 tsp mixed dried herbs (optional)*
- *1 garlic clove, crushed (optional)*
- *1 tsp wholegrain or Dijon mustard*
- *1 tsp honey or maple syrup (optional)*
- *salt and pepper*

Place all the ingredients in a jar, close the lid well and shake. Adjust the flavours to taste.

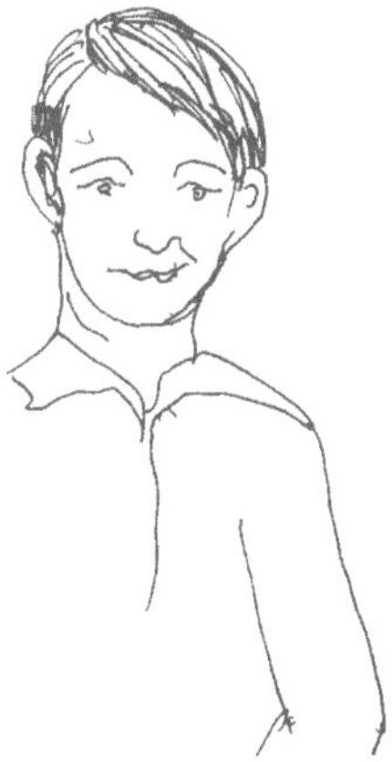

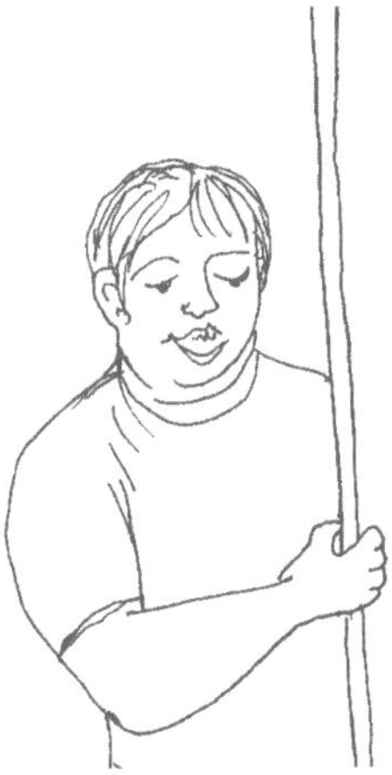

Even the young have type 2 diabetes now. It used to be thought that it was a progressive disease of age. But now it's becoming clear that sugars are to blame.

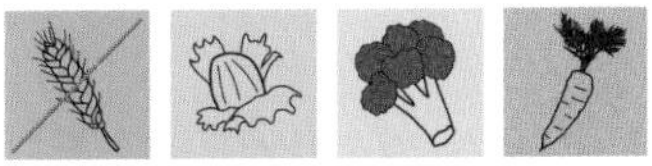

Sweet potato cakes

stove top

serves 4

When compared to normal potatoes, orange sweet potatoes have a higher fibre content, which gives them a low-GI (glycaemic index) and makes them healthier for people with diabetes.

- *1 sweet potato, finely grated*
- *2 garlic cloves, chopped*
- *1 green chilli, chopped*
- *2 coriander sprigs, chopped*
- *1 tbsp soy or tamari sauce*
- *plain gluten-free flour, for shaping*
- *4 tbsp oil, for frying*
- *1 tbsp sesame seeds*

In a bowl, mash together the sweet potatoes, garlic, chilli, coriander and soy or tamari.

On a plate, shape the mixture into little cakes using the flour to prevent it sticking to your hands. Squeeze the patties a little as you form them to free any moisture as you mix with the flour.

Fry the cakes in some oil in a pan on both sides until golden brown, then check if the potato is cooked – if not, fry them for a little longer on each side.

Transfer to a plate lined with kitchen paper to drain off excess oil, then sprinkle with sesame seeds.

Serve while hot and crispy.

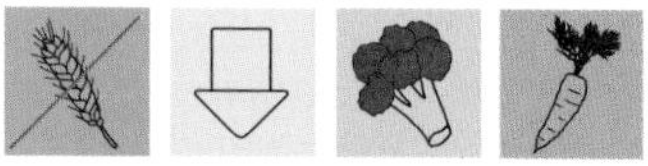

Sweet potato & pumpkin doughnuts

stove top & cool oven

serves 4–6

A sweet-tasting alternative to commercial doughnuts, leave out the sugar and just roll them in cinnamon, if you wish.

- *125g (4½oz) peeled and diced pumpkin or butternut squash*
- *125g (4½oz) peeled and diced sweet potato*
- *1 tsp salt*
- *1 tsp mixed spice*
- *1 tsp instant dried yeast*
- *250g (9oz) gluten-free flour*
- *oil for deep-frying (such as sunflower or coconut)*
- *1 tbsp sugar*
- *1 tsp ground cinnamon*

Boil the pumpkin and sweet potato chunks in a pan of boiling water for 15 minutes, until soft, then drain and mash. Allow to cool.

In a large mixing bowl, combine the salt, spice and yeast, then add the cooled pumpkin and sweet potato mash. Mix well and add enough of the flour to make a soft dough. Cover with a clean tea towel and set aside for 2 hours or until it has doubled in size.

Using floury hands, divide the dough into 20 even pieces (add more flour if necessary), then form them into doughnut shapes and poke a large hole through the middle of each. Leave to rise on a floured baking tray in a warm place for 10–15 minutes.

Meanwhile, heat the oil in a wok or deep-frying pan and set the oven to a low temperature. Deep-fry the doughnuts in batches for 4–5 minutes until golden brown, turning once. Keep the cooked doughnuts in a warm oven until they are all done.

Mix the sugar and cinnamon on a plate and roll the doughnuts in it until they are covered all over, then serve warm.

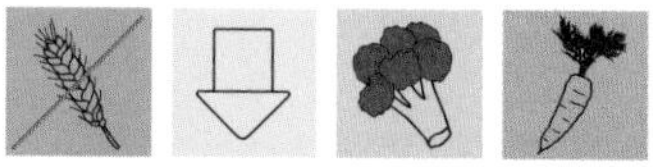

Baked apples

hot oven

per person

Simple but delicious, leave out the sweetness for those with a severe condition or modify to suit.

- *1 juicy medium apple (homegrown or Bramley), cored*
- *2 tbsp filling – a mix of chopped nuts, seeds or raisins*
- *1 tsp maple syrup or honey*
- *½ tsp grated nutmeg or ground cinnamon (optional)*

Heat the oven to 180°C/ fan160°C/350°F/Gas 4. Place the cored apples on an oiled baking tray.

Mix the filling with the maple syrup or honey and spoon it into the centre of each apple. Drift the spice over the top, if using. Bake for 30 minutes or until the apples are soft.

Serve with cream, yogurt or your preferred dairy substitute.

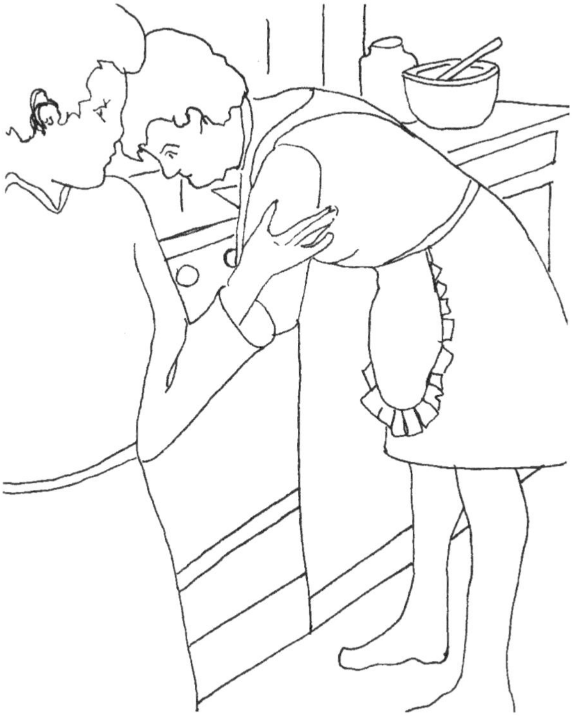

Would you like the recipe
for my sugarless cakes?

No thanks!

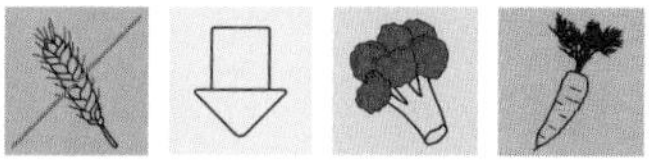

Baked bananas

moderate oven

per person

A good alternative to rich puddings, these are delicious made on a campfire (wrap in foil to bake in the hot ashes).

- *1 banana*
- *1 tsp honey or maple syrup*
- *1 square chocolate (optional)*

Heat the oven to 180°C/ fan160°C/350°F/Gas 4.

Make a slit in the banana skin and spoon in the honey or maple syrup and chocolate, if using. Place on a baking tray and bake for 15 minutes or until the skin is brown and the flesh is soft and translucent.

Cool for 5 minutes, then serve in the skin or spooned out, with ice-cream.

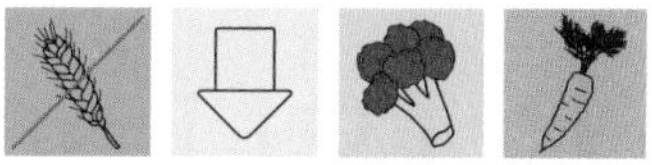

Homemade chocolate

freezer

There are so many chocolate bars available now. This one is cheap to make but tastes expensive and you can adjust the level of sweetness yourself.

- *80g (3oz) cocoa butter or coconut oil*
- *4 tbsp cocoa powder*
- *2 tbsp agave syrup or honey*
- *½ tsp vanilla paste (optional)*
- *pinch of rock salt (optional)*

Line a small flan tray with cling film. Melt the cocoa butter or coconut oil in a bowl set over a pan of simmering water.

Remove the bowl from heat and add the cocoa powder and agave syrup or honey and vanilla paste and salt, if using. Stir with a metal spoon and pour into the prepared tray.

Cover with cling film and freeze for 1 hour before using.

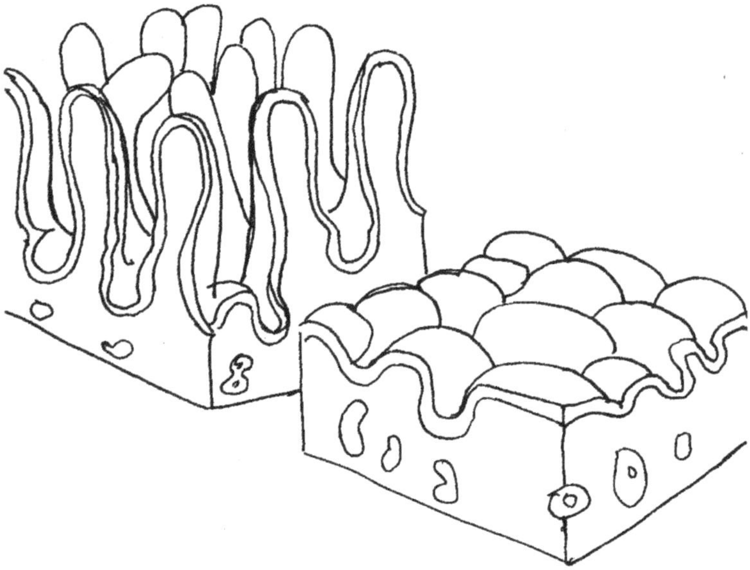

The villi which line the large intestine become severely shortened and flattened in response to gluten in people who are coeliac (right). Left shows normal villi.

GLUTEN INTOLERANCE

Gluten is a protein found in grains such as wheat, barley, rye and oats. There are quite a few gluten-related disorders, ranging from gluten sensitivity to gluten intolerance, coeliac disease and wheat allergy. Non-coeliac gluten sensitivity is a condition that is recognised as a problem across the world.

Coeliac disease is an auto-immune disorder of genetic origin, where the body's immune system attacks itself when gluten is eaten. This causes damage to the lining of the gut and means that nutrients from food cannot be absorbed.

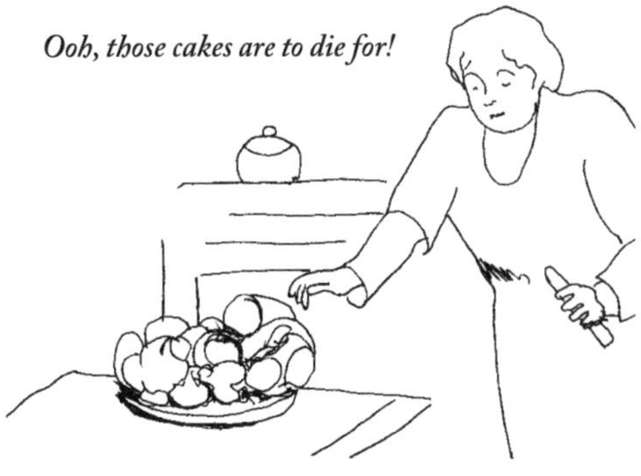

Dylis

Dylis was brought up in an old-fashioned way. She had to clear her plate before leaving the table and eat up her greens. She was not to answer back nor make a fuss, but she kept getting sick and felt pain in her tummy almost every day. Trips to the doctor revealed nothing and she was told she was being naughty and a fusspot.

She was regularly sent to bed and the bedroom door was locked until she could calm down and eat her crusts. She was made to promise to stop crying and screaming and making herself sick.

She says that, like many coeliac children, she was hyperactive, which didn't help people to sympathise with her. She was 50 by the time her diagnosis came through. Even a bite of a mince pie at the work's Christmas do is enough give her symptoms for days after.

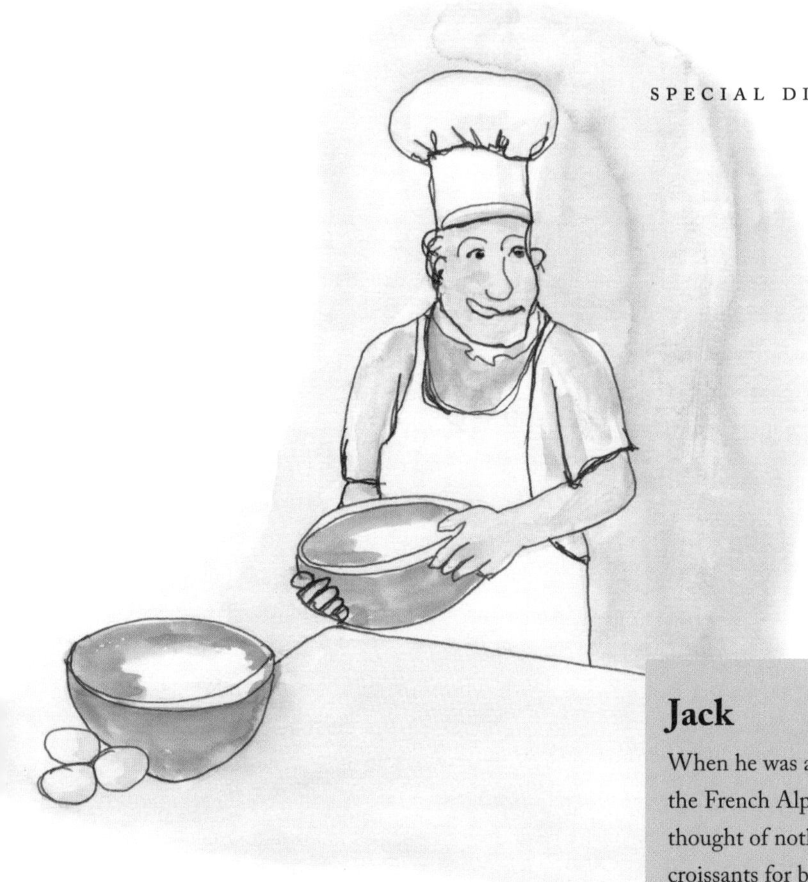

Baking with alternative flours has never been easier.

Wheat allergy is a reaction to proteins found in wheat. It is triggered by the immune system and usually occurs within seconds or minutes of eating. Symptoms of an allergy to wheat can include swelling of the lips and tongue, trouble breathing, itching, hives or anaphylaxis.

Someone with a wheat allergy, but without gluten sensitivity, must avoid eating any form of wheat, but does not have trouble tolerating gluten from non-wheat sources.

While coeliac disease and wheat allergy are well-defined conditions, non-coeliac gluten sensitivity is poorly understood. In non-coeliac gluten sensitivity and intolerance, symptoms similar to, and as severe as, coeliac disease are experienced, but the immune system does not seem to be involved because no antibodies are produced, and there does not appear to be damage to the gut lining. People who are gluten sensitive suffer gastrointestinal symptoms and often have fatigue and headaches as well.

Jack

When he was a teenager Jack was on a climbing trip in the French Alps. He and a friend camped out and thought of nothing but climbing. Every day they had croissants for breakfast and sticks of French bread with lumps of cheese for lunch and for supper too.

They had been there for about four days when Jack awoke with such severe pains that his friend thought he was dying and called an ambulance.

The hospital medics thought he had pancreatitis and wanted to keep him in for observation. His small room was windowless and now that he was on a limited diet, he realised that his mild diarrhoea and constipation problems he'd had since puberty had become grotesquely severe when he had eaten so much marvellous French bread – all those baguettes and pain au chocolat! Besides, now he was feeling so much better. He didn't understand French and felt trapped, so he ran away back to the UK.

At home Jack visited his doctor who suggested a trial for coeliac disease, but he didn't want to go through the pain and decided to self-regulate his intake of gluten instead. He now eats spelt bread and avoids certain beers. His most recent episode of deep pain and bloating was from indulging in too many onion rings with his pub lunch.

People with coeliac disease usually suffer from gastrointestinal symptoms such as cramping, diarrhoea and constipation, as well as bone or joint pain, headaches or fatigue. Coeliac disease, non-coeliac gluten sensitivity and wheat allergy are conditions that can be treated with the appropriate diet and with the elimination of either gluten or wheat.

Rebecca

Rebecca did not know for many years that she had a problem with wheat gluten. Eventually her osteopath recommended an exclusion diet to see if that might help her symptoms.

Rebecca says, 'In my 30s I was a working mum, with a full-time job in London and two school-aged children. I was tired all the time but then that wasn't surprising; my job was all-consuming, my children and home were demanding. We ate what the children favoured – a diet heavily predicated on Anglo-Italian menus, such as pasta, pizza and then more pasta. We would gulp down our Weetabix in the morning before running off in various directions, then I would grab a sandwich at my desk so I could leave the office on time in the evening.

'Despite regular exercise I got larger and was struggling with back pain. On the exclusion diet I cut out everything except unprocessed fruit and vegetables and kept this up for a week. Alcohol was the first thing to creep back in (closely followed by coffee the next morning). Back came the dairy, though I never got used to putting cow juice in my tea again. Then came my first bite of a slice of bread and I knew what the culprit was. My stomach filled with gas almost immediately and later my joints began to ache.'

That was over 20 years ago. Now Rebecca is lucky to be able to tolerate oats and spelt, which makes life easier, though one bite of gluten-rich wheat will cause her to develop mouth ulcers, nausea and bloating.

I know several people who have gluten sensitivity who can eat and tolerate sourdough bread made from original varieties of wheat such as spelt, essene and emmer.

Adam

I met Adam on a course and invited him to visit. He was a young writer and needed somewhere to stay occasionally to get on with editing his dystopian novel. He came for a few days and seemed quite happy at first, helping in the garden, going for walks and writing in his room.

We had pizza the first night and homemade quiche for lunch next day. On the third morning, he looked decidedly grumpy and went straight back to his room, refusing the toast that was on offer for breakfast.

Odder still, he stayed in his room till lunchtime. At lunch, I asked if he was okay and commented on his behaviour in a mild way, whereupon he broke down and confessed that he had a gluten intolerance and said he had not wanted to make a fuss by telling us but was now feeling terrible.

He then said he had not even told his parents and suffered every time he went to visit them, but he couldn't tell them for fear of them teasing him and not understanding how much it affected him.

We had soup and rye crackers for lunch and afterwards went shopping so he could buy all the foodstuff he needed, and he relaxed, a lot.

Adam still comes to visit us. He is now editing the prequel to what became a series of novels. He told his family about his reaction to gluten and, of course, they did not laugh at him.

Beetroot & goat's cheese tart

moderate oven

serves 4

This is a sumptuous flan, good enough to serve at a celebratory dinner. Gluten free pastry is difficult to make but good GF readymade pastry such as Genius is available or try the recipe on page 78. As a variation, substitute feta for goat's cheese.

- *1 x 22cm (9in) bought gluten-free pastry case or readymade pastry*
- *3 small red onions, finely chopped*
- *25g (1oz) olive oil or butter*
- *450g (1lb) beetroot wedges, boiled and peeled*
- *2 tbsp cider vinegar*
- *1½ tbsp honey*
- *150ml (5fl oz) liquid (water or red wine)*
- *1 tsp thyme leaves*
- *280g (10oz) goat's cheese roll, sliced*
- *salt and pepper*

Heat the oven to 200°C/ fan180°C/400°F/Gas 6. Put the pastry case in a flan tin or on a baking sheet.

Sauté the onions in a pan with the oil or butter until they are soft. Tip out onto a plate and set to one side. In the same pan, sauté the cooked beetroot. Stir in the vinegar and honey, season to taste and fry for 2 minutes until most of it has been absorbed. Add the water or red wine, onions and thyme and simmer until most of the liquid has been absorbed.

Lay half the goat's cheese in the base of the pastry case. Cover with the beetroot mix and lay the rest of the cheese on top.

Bake in the oven for 20–30 minutes until the cheese is bubbling and turning golden. Cool a little before serving.

Gram flour patties

stove top

serves 4

Make these in minutes for an unexpected lunch guest or as a hot snack for children who cannot have regular flour products.

- *110g (4oz) gram flour*
- *½ tsp bicarbonate of soda (baking soda)*
- *1 tsp curry powder*
- *½ tsp ground turmeric*
- *100ml (3½fl oz) water*
- *3 tbsps mix of thinly sliced courgettes (zucchini), red pepper, mushroom, onion*
- *110g (4oz) feta, cut into small cubes*
- *1 tsp chopped coriander (cilantro) leaves*
- *oil, for shallow frying*
- *salt and pepper*

Mix the gram flour with the bicarbonate of soda, seasoning and spices in a large bowl. Add the water and stir into a smooth, dropping consistency. Add the rest of the ingredients and mix well.

Heat the oil in a frying pan until hot and then add spoonfuls of the patty mix to the hot oil and fry in batches until golden brown on both sides.

Serve immediately.

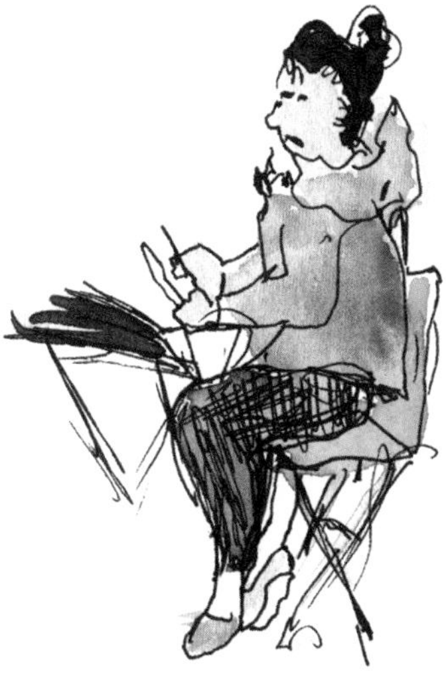

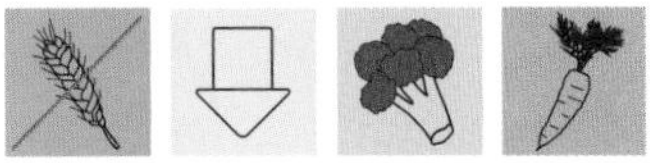

Gluten-free pastry

oven

serves 4

Take time to perfect your recipe for GF pastry which can sometimes be over crispy or cardboard like. This is a good beginning. To make sweet pastry add 25g (1oz) sugar and 1 teaspoon of vanilla essence.

- *75g (3oz) gluten-free flour*
- *75g (3oz) buckwheat flour*
- *½ tsp xanthan gum (optional)*
- *60g (2oz) vegan fat*
- *2 tbsp cold water*
- *salt and pepper*
- *22cm (9in) pie tin*

Combine the flours, salt, xanthan gum and seasoning in a large mixing bowl. Rub the fat into the flour mix until it resembles breadcrumbs. Add the cold water by the spoonful, until there is a binding dough. Wrap the dough in cling film and place in the fridge for 30 minutes.

Heat the oven to 200°C/ fan180°C/400°F/Gas 6.

Roll out the pastry gently between two sheets of greaseproof paper until it is about 12mm (½in) thick. Strip away one sheet of greaseproof paper and carefully transfer the pastry to a 22cm (9in) pie tin for baking. Make good any breaks. Pastry made with gluten-free flour can be tough if not treated very gently.

Blind bake the pastry. Line the pie tin with baking parchment and fill with ceramic baking beans or dried pulses. Bake for 10 minutes then remove the beans and baking parchment and cook for 5 minutes more until golden brown. Allow to cool for a minute or two before adding any filling.

Homemade pies

These pies can be made at the same time, for the same meal by doubling up on the vegetable ingredients.

- **Use vegan pastry for all (purchase gluten-free pastry if needed).**
- **Cook the vegetables for all pies at the same time. Make the vegan pie and set aside vegetables for the meat version.**
- **Make the vegan / gluten-free pie and set aside. Keep it warm but separate by wrapping it in clean tea towel until ready to serve.**
- **Fry the meat and make the meat pie.**
- **Use clean serving tools for vegan version.**

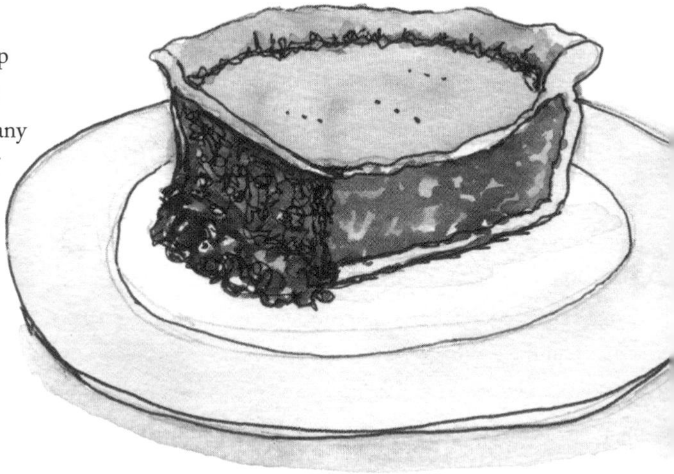

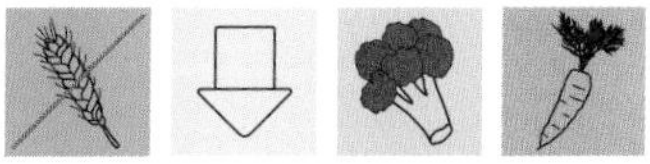

Leek & potato pie

oven

serves 4

Use the GF pastry recipe (see page 78) or buy readymade without too many additives.

- *450g (1lb) small potatoes, quartered*
- *2 onions, finely chopped*
- *450g (1lb) leeks, cut into 2cm (¾in) rings*
- *2 tbsp olive oil*
- *5 tbsp water, stock or soya cream*
- *1 tbsp vegan bouillon liquid (optional)*
- *1 tbsp dried rosemary*
- *enough gluten-free pastry for 1 x 22cm (9in) pastry case and a lid (see page 78)*
- *a little nut milk to glaze*
- *salt and pepper*

Boil the potatoes in a large pan of water until just soft and then drain.

Sauté the onions and leeks in a frying pan in the olive oil until they are soft and golden. Stir the onions and leeks into potatoes and add the liquid. Season well, add the ːmary and set to one side while you prepare the base.

Ieat the oven to 180°C/ fan160°C/350°F/Gas 4. Grease ʔcm (9in) pie tin or pie dish.

ɾoll out the pastry and line the greased pie dish. Blind .e for 10 minutes (see page 78). Let the pastry cool for a ıute or two but leave the oven on. Fill the case with the led mix and make a lid of the rest of the pastry, ching to close the rim. Brush the top with nut milk.

Ͻook in the centre of the oven for 20–30 minutes until med through and the pastry lid is cooked to golden.

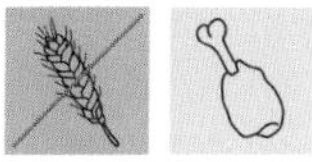

Meat & potato pie

oven

serves 4

Use the GF pastry recipe (see page 78) or buy readymade without too many additives. Make this alongside and separately from the leek and potato for a mixed feast. Use this recipe to make individual small pies in a muffin tray for picnics or a cold lunch.

- *450g (1lb) small potatoes, quartered*
- *2 tbsp olive oil*
- *2 onions, finely chopped*
- *250g (8oz) leeks, cut into 2cm rings*
- *1 tbsp olive oil*
- *250g (8oz) minced lamb or beef*
- *5 tbsp water or stock*
- *1 tbsp vegan bouillon liquid (optional)*
- *1 tbsp dried rosemary*
- *enough gluten-free pastry for 1 x 22cm (9in) pastry case and a lid (see page 78)*
- *1 beaten egg, to glaze*
- *salt and pepper*

Boil the potatoes in a large pan of water until just soft and then drain.

Sauté the onions and leeks in a frying pan in the olive oil until they are soft and golden.

Fry the mince in the saucepan in the oil until browned. Use the fat to re-fry the vegetables, adding the liquid and bouillon to make a thin gravy and mix together with the rosemary and seasoning. Set to one side while you prepare the base.

Heat the oven to 180°C/ fan160°C/350°F/Gas 4. Grease a 22cm (9in) pie dish.

Roll out the pastry and line the greased pie dish. Blind bake for 10 minutes (see page 78). Let the pastry cool for a minute or two but leave the oven on. Fill the case with the cooled mix and make a lid of the rest of the pastry, pinching to close the rim. Brush the top with the beaten egg.

Cook in the centre of the oven for 20–30 minutes until warmed through and the pastry lid is cooked to golden.

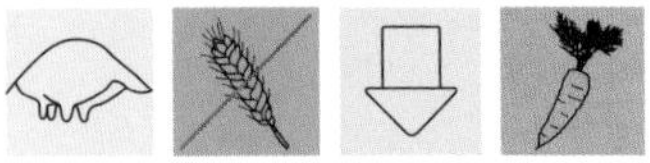

Squash, spinach & goat's cheese pie

stove top & moderate oven

serves 4

Use the GF pastry recipe (see page 78) or buy readymade. Stirring 1 tablespoon of vegan bouillon in with the spinach will give a richer taste to the vegan version. You can adapt this recipe to make individual small pies for picnics and if you want a vegan version, just leave out the cheese and egg.

- *450g (1lb) butternut squash, peeled and cut into 1–2cm (¼in – ½in) cubes*
- *2 carrots, chopped*
- *2 medium onions, finely sliced*
- *2 garlic cloves, pressed*
- *2 tbsp olive oil*
- *125g (4½oz) spinach, finely chopped*
- *125g (4½oz) goat's cheese*
- *1 tbsp chopped rosemary or sage (optional)*
- *1 tsp tamari sauce (optional)*
- *enough gluten-free pastry for 1 x 22cm (9in) pastry case and a lid (see page 78)*
- *a little nut milk or 1 beaten egg, to glaze*
- *salt and pepper*

Steam the squash and carrots for 7–10 minutes or until soft.

Sauté the onions and garlic in a frying pan in the olive oil and season well.

Combine all the vegetables and stir in the spinach. Add the goat's cheese or herbs and sprinkle with tamari, if using. Set to one side to cool while you prepare the base.

Heat the oven to 180°C/ fan160°C/350°F/Gas 4. Grease a 22cm (9in) pie dish.

Line a pie dish with half the pastry and blind bake for 10 minutes (see page 78). Let the pastry cool for a minute or two but leave the oven on. Fill the case with the cooled mix and make a lid with the rest of the pastry, pinching to close the rim. Brush the top with milk substitute or brush with a beaten egg.

Cook in the oven for 20–30 minutes until warmed through and the pastry is cooked.

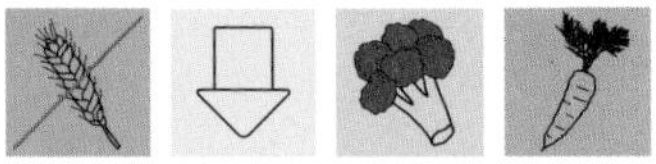

Gluten-free pizza base

oven

makes 2 pizza bases

We use this to cook pizza at home. It makes a generous base whether for the electric or the wood-fired oven. Try cooking the base a little before topping for a crisper finish.

- *125g (4½oz) buckwheat flour, plus extra for dusting*
- *125g (4½oz) quinoa flour*
- *1 tsp instant dried yeast*
- *1 tsp sugar*
- *1 tsp salt*
- *300ml (10fl oz) warm water*
- *2 tbsp olive oil*

In a bowl, combine the dry ingredients. Mix together the water and oil and knead into the dry mix. Add more water if the mix is too dry, more buckwheat if too wet. The dough should be soft and pliable.

Divide the dough evenly into 2 balls and roll out each on a well-floured board. If the pastry is too fragile, roll it between two pieces of baking paper.

Transfer to a pizza stone or baking sheet and allow to rise a little before topping and cooking.

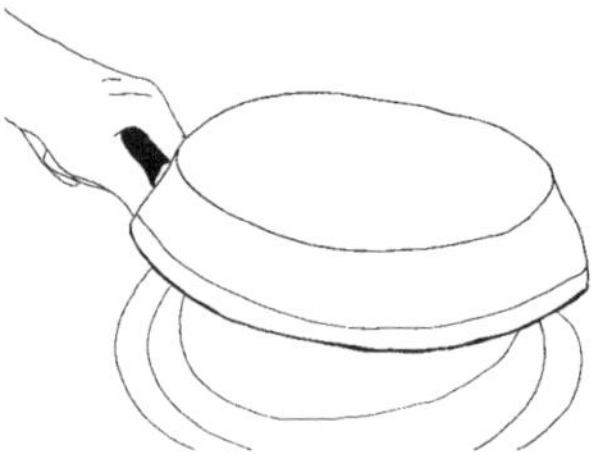

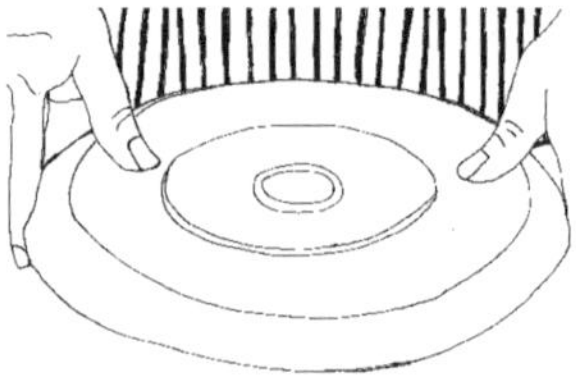

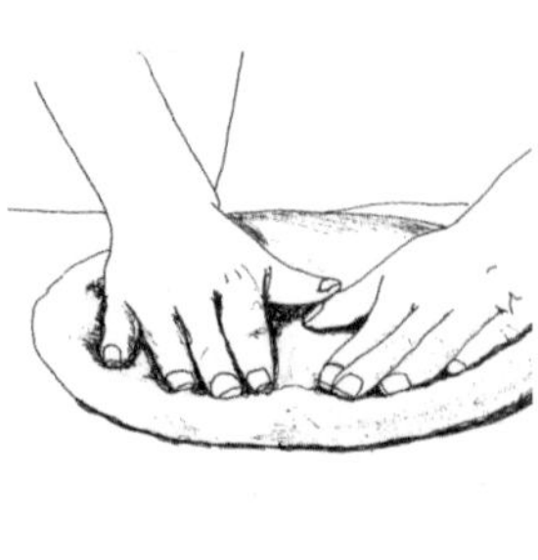

Grain & nut-free pizza base

stove top & oven

per person

For people who cannot tolerate grains or nuts as well as being gluten free this is a little wonder. At last they can eat pizza! Replace the egg by making a flax egg by mixing one tablespoon of ground flaxseeds with three tablespoons of water. Leave in the fridge for 15–30 minutes until it has thickened. You can use the grated cauliflower as a rice to accompany curries, too.

- *1 medium cauliflower*
- *1 tbsp egg or egg substitute*
- *1 tsp dried vegan bouillon*
- *1 tsp dried oregano*
- *1 tsp dried basil*
- *1 garlic clove, minced*
- *1 tbsp cornflour*
- *oil, for frying*
- *salt and pepper*

Either blend or grate the cauliflower so it resembles rice grains. Place the cauliflower 'rice' in a saucepan and cover with boiling water to simmer for 2 minutes. Drain the cauliflower 'rice' through a sieve and squeeze it to remove as much liquid as you can.

Allow to cool and add the flax egg or egg, seasoning, bouillon, herbs, garlic and cornflour to the drained cauliflower. Mix until it all sticks together.

Lightly oil a heavy frying pan or skillet and spread enough dough to fill a circle 5–7mm (¼in) thick and slightly thicker at the edge. Fry slowly for 3–5 minutes until it is golden and crusty.

Flip it onto the other side using a plate and fry for 3–4 minutes more. It will be crusty on the outside and softer in the middle.

Then flip the base onto the pizza peel or baking sheet, add your toppings and cook in the usual way – don't overload it, though, as too much sauce can make the crust soggy.

Gluten-free focaccia flatbread

oven

I first made this for a wedding when it surpassed my expectations. When it is fresh it is truly yummy.

- *250g (9oz) gluten-free flour*
- *1 tsp instant dried yeast*
- *½ tsp xanthan gum*
- *1 tsp sea salt*
- *1 tsp sugar*
- *100ml (3½fl oz) warm milk substitute*
- *2 tbsp extra virgin olive oil, plus extra for greasing*
- *2 tbsp aquafaba (the briny water in tins of chickpeas, see page 134)*
- *¼ tsp bicarbonate of soda (baking soda)*
- *2 tsp white wine vinegar*

Topping

- *1 tbsp olive oil, plus extra for greasing*
- *1 tbsp sliced olives*
- *1 tbsp fresh rosemary leaves*
- *½ tsp sea salt flakes*

Sift together the flour, yeast, xanthan gum and salt into a large mixing bowl.

Mix the sugar and milk substitute together in a bowl, add the oil and aquafaba and beat together. Beat into the flour mix to make a soft dough.

Mix the bicarbonate of soda and white vinegar together to fizz, then fold into the mixture.

Using oiled hands, smooth the dough out into an oiled baking tray. Cover and keep in a warm place for 45 minutes or so to rise until puffy.

Heat the oven to 190°C/ fan170°C/375°F/Gas 5.

Once the bread has doubled in size, poke holes into the dough to make indentations. Drizzle with the olive oil and sprinkle with olives, rosemary leaves and the sea salt flakes. Bake for 30 minutes until the top is golden.

This is best eaten when fresh.

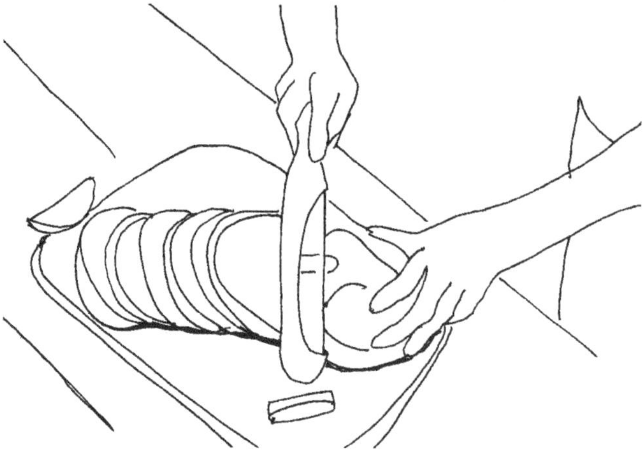

Homemade rye bread

oven

makes 2 small loaves

When you are used to using sourdough starter you can substitute it for the yeast to make this even nicer. Add a tablespoon of caraway seed for extra flavour. Lighten this heavy bread by substituting a third of spelt, white rye or gluten-free flour instead of all rye. Good for toasting, this bread usually has a crispy crust and a doughy centre.

- *2 tsp instant dried yeast*
- *300g (10oz) gluten-free rye flour*
- *1 tsp salt*
- *1 tbsp molasses or brown sugar (optional)*
- *250ml (8fl oz) warm water*
- *oil, for greasing*

Combine all the dry ingredients in a large bowl.

Add the molasses or sugar to the water, if using, and pour into the flour mix. Work with a wooden spoon to make a smooth, soft dough.

Grease two small bread tins with oil and divide the dough between them. Smooth the tops with a wet spatula. Cover with a cloth and leave in a warm place for several hours until the dough doubles in size.

Heat the oven to 190°C/ fan170°C/375°F/Gas 5. Bake for about 40 minutes or until it sounds hollow when tapped on the underside. Cool on a wire rack.

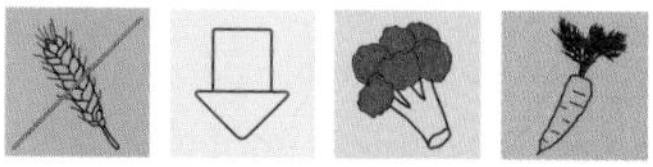

Gluten-free bread

oven

makes 1 loaf

This makes a lighter loaf than the rye bread but still heavier and more 'artisanal' than the average white loaf.

- *110g (4oz) buckwheat kernels*
- *50g (2oz) hulled millet*
- *1 tbsp psyllium husk*
- *1 tbsp poppy seeds*
- *1 tbsp quick yeast*
- *1 tsp salt*
- *2 tsp xanthan gum*
- *140g (5oz) arrowroot*
- *225g (8oz) rice flour*
- *400ml (14fl oz) warm water*
- *3 tbsp oil, plus 1 tsp oil for greasing*
- *1 tbsp rice or maple syrup*

Grind the buckwheat and millet for a few seconds to break up the seeds but not turn them into a powder. Add them to a mixing bowl with all the other dry ingredients.

To the warm water, add the oil and syrup, mix it into the dry ingredients and knead for a few minutes. Oil a bread tin, put in the mix and round off the top. Brush water on the top of the loaf and leave to rise. Check occasionally to see if it needs rewetting. This will assist the rise.

Heat the oven to 180°C/ fan160°C/350°F/Gas 4.

Bake for about 1 hour, until done and the top is golden then remove from the tin to cool on a rack.

Churros

stove top

serves 4–6

Delicious to the point of decadence, these churros are almost like old-fashioned fairground doughnuts but completely gluten free.

- *3 tbsp water*
- *1 tbsp sugar, plus 1 tbsp for coating*
- *½ tsp salt*
- *2 tbsp sunflower oil*
- *110g (4oz) gluten-free flour*
- *oil, for deep-frying*
- *1 tsp ground cinnamon*

Combine the first four ingredients in a saucepan and bring to the boil. Remove from the heat and stir in enough flour to form a soft dough.

Heat the oil and drop a spoonful of mix into it – if it sizzles it is hot enough. Drop spoonfuls into the hot oil in batches or fill an icing bag with the mix and squeeze out in 4cm (1½in) lengths into the oil. Fry the churros until golden all over.

Drain and roll in the sugar and cinnamon before serving, or drizzle with chocolate sauce (see below).

Chocolate sauce for churros

stove top

serves 4–6

This very simple recipe makes a chocolate sauce that can be used on churros (see above) or poured over ice-cream and other desserts like fried bananas.

- *120g (4½oz) sugar*
- *55g (2oz) cocoa powder*
- *100ml (3½fl oz) water*
- *1 tsp vanilla paste*

Mix the sugar and cocoa powder together in a saucepan, then add a little water and stir to form a paste. Pour in the rest of the water and heat to boiling.

Remove from the heat and stir in the vanilla paste. Simmer for 2 minutes.

Serve hot over churros or ice-cream.

Gluten-free hot cross buns

oven

makes 12

The joy of joining in and eating hot cross buns whenever everyone else is tucking in on Good Friday morning or any other morning! These are soft and fully ready to toast.

- *300g (10oz) gluten-free flour OR 150g (5oz) cassava flour and 150g (5oz) buckwheat flour*
- *1 tsp salt*
- *1 tsp ground nutmeg or cinnamon*
- *1 tsp instant dried yeast*
- *200g (7oz) dried apricots, roughly chopped*
- *1 tbsp maple syrup*
- *300ml (10fl oz) warm water*

For best results use a silicon muffin tray.

In a mixing bowl, combine the dry ingredients and apricots.

Mix the maple syrup with the warm water and add it slowly to the dry ingredients. Use enough to make a soft dough.

Spoon the dough into the muffin tray and brush a little water over the top of each.

Crosses

Make a soft pastry from the buckwheat flour and water. Roll this to a flat floured sheet and cut strips to make the crosses. Use a dab of water to fix the strips cross ways on the buns. Leave to rise until doubled in size.

Heat the oven to 180°C/ fan160°C/350°F/Gas 4. Bake for 20–30 minutes or until the bun part is golden brown. Remove from the tray and cool on a rack. These are best eaten split in half and toasted.

Maltitol is a polyol.

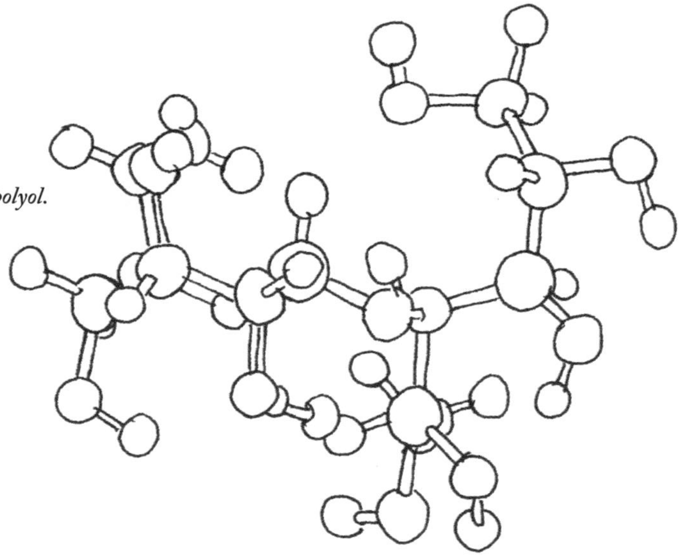

FODMAP

FODMAP is an acronym of Fermentable Oligosaccharides, Disaccharides, Monosaccharides and Polyols – which are osmotically active, rapidly fermentable, short-chain carbohydrates. These are mostly plant-based carbohydrates that some people, such as those with IBS, do not digest very well, and because FODMAPs aren't absorbed in the gut, they begin to ferment in the large intestine, causing bloating and gas. This results in pain, flatulence and diarrhoea.

FODMAP carbohydrates, such as polyols (P), can be made in a laboratory. Some polyols occur naturally as sugars in beetroot and fruits like peaches and plums, but many are manufactured from corn syrup. These have E numbers and can carry a warning that they may cause diarrhoea. An example of a wholly manufactured polyol is maltitol. Maltitol is manufactured by hydrogenating maltose, a naturally occurring disaccharide, which is derived from cornflour. It is a highly attractive sugar replacement, as maltitol is 90 per cent as sweet as sugar. Its food additive number is E965.

Everyone needs carbohydrates in one form or another – we even have an enzyme in our saliva that breaks down cooked starch. But not all carbohydrates are good for us all the time, so when your gut biome is compromised, you may be encouraged to try a FODMAP diet.

The FODMAP diet is a short-term elimination diet designed by Australian nutritionists to alleviate the symptoms of IBS. The strict diet is intended to last for six weeks, which is felt to be enough time for the gut biome to re-establish itself. High-FODMAP foods are then re-introduced one at a time. Not everyone will have a problem with every FODMAP; some might have symptoms triggered by one or two types of FODMAPs, whereas others may be sensitive to all five. The diet is intended to be individualised according to the problematic FODMAP, so people are advised to see a dietician.

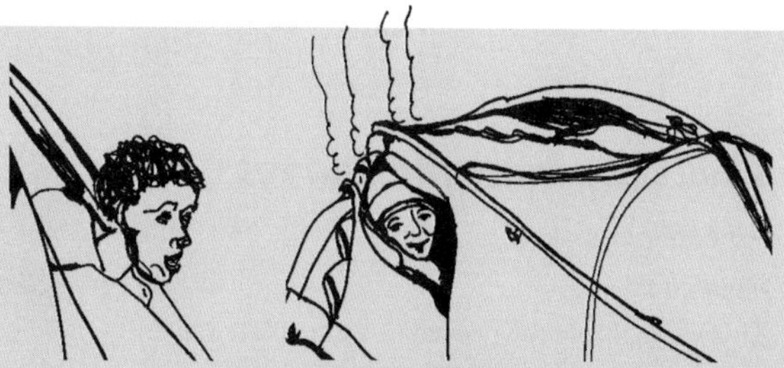

Phoawh! Someone un-zip the tent!

Sue

I first learned of the FODMAP diet from Sue, a young friend with a very active lifestyle. After a camping trip, Sue found she had a tick bite and then flu-like symptoms, which turned out to be Lyme disease. After several bouts of antibiotics to cure the Lyme disease, Sue pretty much recovered but was left with Irritable Bowel Syndrome (IBS)-type symptoms of bloating and diarrhoea. She was recommended to go on a FODMAP diet to help re-establish her gut biome. Now she is back to normal and almost as energetic as she once was.

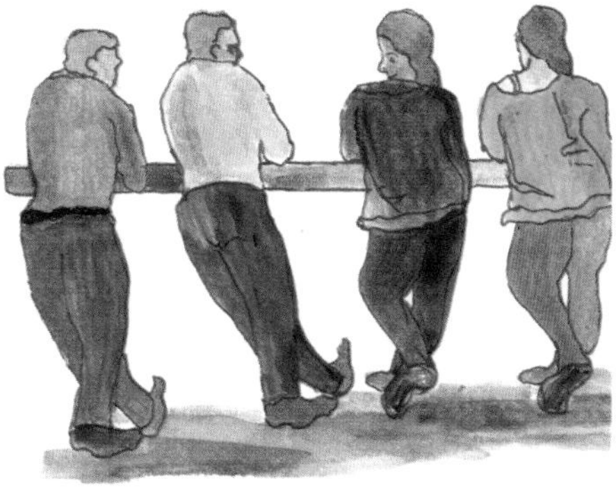

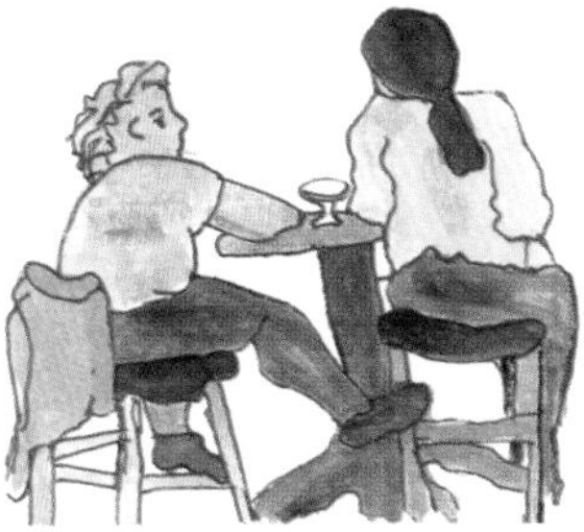

FODMAPs are not foods to be avoided unless you have symptoms of IBS, diverticulitis or suffer from excessive bloating and wind on a regular basis. Many of the carbohydrates in FODMAPs are useful for the body and the gut. For instance, besides being component parts of many plants (which we use as dietary fibre), oligosaccharides play an important role in the way the body recognises and defends against bacteria and viruses whose surface proteins are coated with various oligosaccharides.

Following a FODMAP diet can be difficult socially as there are so many foods that are excluded. So, if you are intending to make a meal for someone on a FODMAP diet it would be good to ask them what they can eat rather than what they can't.

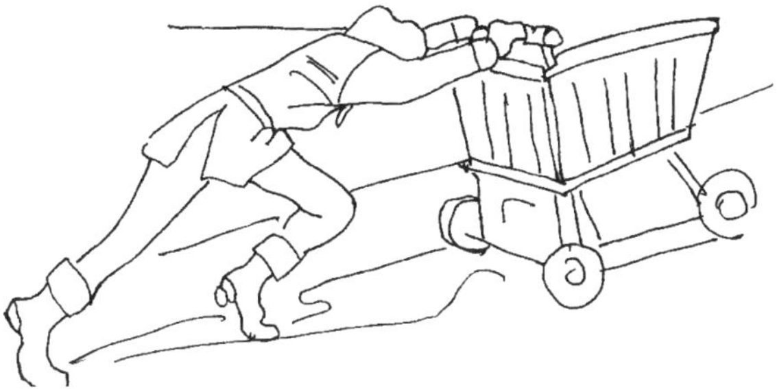

Constipation is an uphill struggle. For many people with IBS, constipation is caused by the fermentation of high-FODMAP foods as they sit in the large intestine.

Heather

At a house party in the countryside, I shared a small table with Heather and Joe. Most people were eating curry, but Heather's plate had only salad and plain rice. Joe sidled up to her and slipped a small package into her hand. She smiled an apology as she drew a small mackerel from the pack and put it on her plate.

Heather was on the FODMAP diet but confessed to feeling shy about dealing with it. She said that as a GP she had been recommending elimination diets of various kinds for years. She told me that she treated many people with digestive difficulties and abdominal symptoms. Before going on a family boat trip, she finally had had to recognise her own health issues and take some drastic measures to deal with acid reflux, bloating and terrible-smelling flatulence.

She had been on the FODMAP diet for over six weeks and was slowly beginning to reintroduce foods and to recognise which foods brought on bloating.

The house party was a challenge because there was so much yummy food on offer and not much choice for anyone who was gastro-divergent or restricting their food groups. She was afraid there would not be much sympathy either, hence hiding the fish.

I asked Heather if she had noticed any mood changes since being on the FODMAP diet and she said she had always had mood swings but that she was feeling more settled. She also said her body was responding very quickly to any food that caused her symptoms, which was both a good and a bad thing, depending on the circumstances.

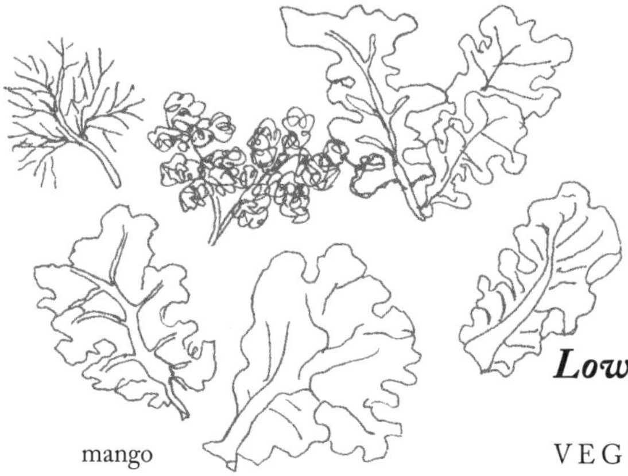

High-Fodmap Foods

VEGETABLES

asparagus, artichokes, avocado

beans, inc. soya, broad beans, haricot, beetroot, broccoli, Brussels sprouts

cabbage (red)

cauliflower

celery

chickpeas

fennel bulb (has high levels of prebiotics but is high FODMAP in a 1–2 cup serving)

fennel seed (in tea)

garlic

leek

onions

mushrooms (most types)

peas

spring onions (white bit)

FRUITS

apples

apricot

avocado

ripe bananas

blackberries

cherries

dates

grapefruit

mango

nectarines

peaches

pears

plums

prunes

raisins

sultanas

NUTS & SEEDS

cashew

pistachio

BAKING INGREDIENTS

agave

desiccated coconut

cornflakes

date syrup

gram flour

kombucha

kefir

molasses

soya milk and yoghurt

teff flour

Low-Fodmap Foods

VEGETABLES

alfalfa

aubergine (eggplant)

bamboo shoots

beansprouts

carrots

celeriac

chard

chickpeas (tinned)

chillies

Chinese greens

courgettes (zucchini)

cucumber

edamame beans

endive

Florence fennel or bulb (in a ½ cup serving)

green beans

ginger

galangal

kale

lettuce

mangetout

mushrooms (shimeji, oyster)

okra

olives

pak choi

parsnip

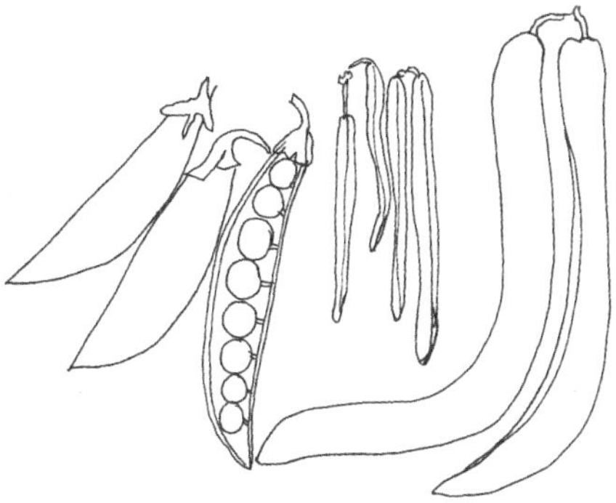

peppers

potato

pumpkin (squash, butternut)

radish

rocket (arugula)

seaweed

spinach

spring onion (green part)

sweet corn

sweet potato

tomatoes

turnip

water chestnuts

yam

NON-VEGAN

any lean, plain meat

eggs

non-fatty fish

lactose-free milk products such as aged cheeses and some yogurts

FRUITS

greener bananas

blueberries

coconut

grapes

kiwi fruit

lemon, lime

mandarin

melon (cantaloupe, rock melon, honeydew)

orange

papaya

passion fruit

pineapple

raspberries

rhubarb

strawberries

SEEDS & NUTS

almonds

chestnuts

hazelnuts

macadamia

pecan

pine-nuts

seeds –

- chia
- linseed
- poppy seeds
- pumpkin seeds
- sesame seeds
- sunflower seeds

BAKING INGREDIENTS

almond milk

agar agar

almond flour

arrowroot

bread (authentically made sourdough bread)

cane sugar

chocolate

cocoa

cornflour

gluten-free flour

hemp milk

maple syrup

miso

peanut butter

popcorn

rice

stevia

tapioca

tofu (traditionally made)

wasabi

yeast extract

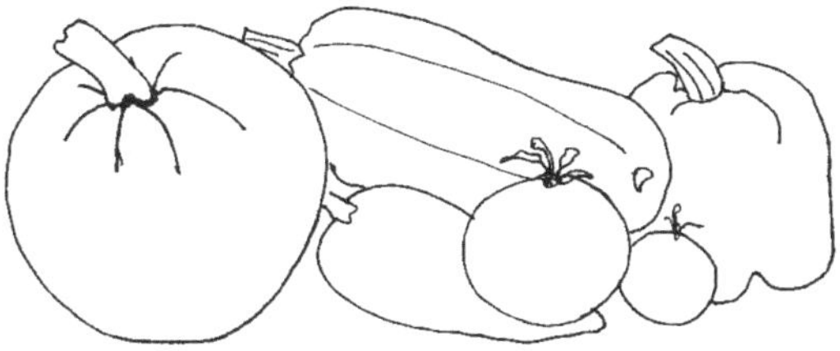

I haven't included many recipes specifically for a FODMAP diet as it is best to ask what a person can eat, but here are a few suggestions for FODMAP meals.

Savoury

- stir-fry and rice
- pad Thai and rice noodles
- satay and rice
- maple and ginger-glazed tempeh
- lemongrass, coconut tofu Thai soup
- quinoa, grated carrot patties
- onion-free ratatouille
- carrot and courgette (zucchini) fritters
- courgette (zucchini) risotto
- fried ginger aubergines (eggplant)
- stuffed courgette (zucchini), peppers or tomatoes
- gluten-free pasta and sauce or lasagne
- roast potatoes
- carrot soup
- savoury no-cheese sauce
- steamed veg and rice or quinoa
- polenta and tomato sauce
- sushi and rice with fish

Puddings & cakes

- gluten-free flour pancakes
- gluten-free flour rhubarb crumble
- lemon and lime sorbet
- polenta cake
- gluten-free biscuits
- sponge cake
- popcorn with salt or sugar
- rice pudding

Amelia

At a community dinner I was sitting opposite lovely Amelia, who was twenty but looked fifteen. She said that she has recently been told that changing her diet could be a way to tackle her psoriasis. When Amelia was a child, she had had bad eczema but that was gone by the time she was seven. When she was thirteen, she had a terrible toothache and root abscess which was treated with long-term antibiotics. Not long afterwards she began to get psoriasis. Her psoriasis disappeared last year when she spent the winter in New Zealand, but this winter it was really affecting her. She pulled up her sleeve to reveal a large burgundy splash across the back of her forearm and elbow. She pointed to the little patches of pink on her face and said, 'I don't mind it so much, except for on my face.'

I suggested that she could ask her doctor about the FODMAP diet, to adjust her gut biome.

As soon as I mentioned fructose as a potential culprit, she laughed and exclaimed, 'But I love fruit. I'm basically addicted to it!'

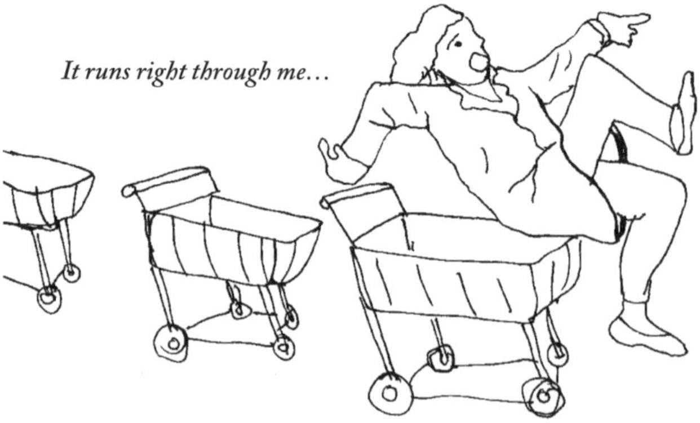

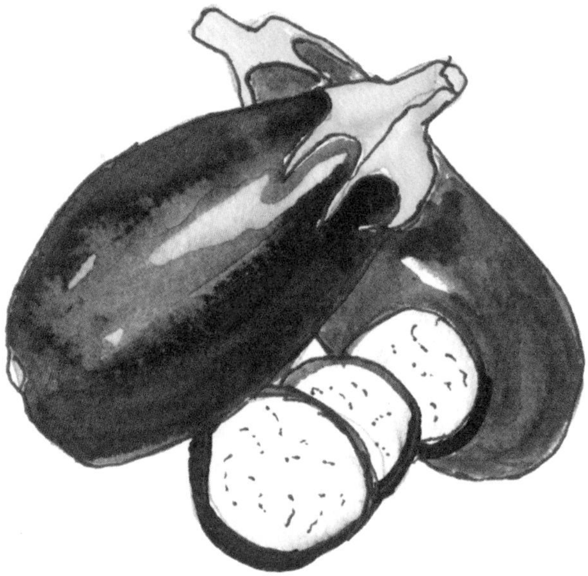

Baba ganoush

moderate oven / barbeque

serves 4

Aubergines are super tasty and low FODMAP. Baba ganoush can be made with aubergines baked until soft, in a hot oven or over hot barbecue coals.

- *1 medium aubergine (eggplant)*
- *1 tbsp lemon juice*
- *1 tbsp tahini*
- *1 garlic clove, minced*
- *1 tbsp olive oil*
- *1 tsp finely chopped coriander (cilantro) or parsley (optional)*
- *salt and pepper*

Heat the oven to 180°C/ fan160°C/350°F/Gas 4. Prick the aubergine a few times with a fork, then place on a baking tray and roast in the oven for 1 hour or until soft (this is convenient to do when baking bread).

Remove from the oven and leave to cool. Scoop out the flesh from the aubergine, discarding the skin. In a small blender, mix the aubergine with the lemon juice, tahini, garlic and oil until it is creamy and smooth.

Season to taste and garnish with chopped coriander and parsley.

Celeriac & salted lemon salad

serves 4

As well as being low FODMAP, celeriac is rich in antioxidants and nutrients, improves digestion and is good for your heart.

- *2 tsp olive oil*
- *2 tsp balsamic or cider vinegar*
- *1 small celeriac, cubed*
- *2 quarters salted lemons, finely chopped (see page 69)*
- *2 spring onions, finely chopped*
- *1 tsp coriander seeds*
- *1 tsp thyme leaves, finely chopped*
- *125g (4oz) feta cheese, cut into cubes (optional)*
- *1 tbsp finely chopped parsley leaves*
- *salt and pepper*

Make a dressing by combining the oil and vinegar in a bowl.

Place the celeriac cubes in a steamer and steam for 12 minutes or until soft. Drain and allow to cool.

In a large salad bowl, mix all the ingredients together, pour on the dressing, toss and season to taste. Set aside for an hour to allow it to mellow before serving.

Aubergine stuffed with itself

moderate oven

per person

This is a hearty dish which is simple to make using low FODMAP ingredients.

- *1 aubergine (eggplant)*
- *1 tbsp olive oil*
- *225g (8oz) cooked or tinned red or green lentils*
- *1 tsp herbs or spices to taste (try mixed herbs or mild curry powder)*
- *topping of sesame seeds, breadcrumbs or cheese (something crispy or crumbly)*
- *salt and pepper*

Heat the oven to 180°C/ fan160°C/350°F/Gas 4.

Cut the aubergine in half and scoop out the flesh, keeping the rind and ½cm of flesh all round. Dice the removed flesh. Fry the diced flesh in a pan with half the olive oil until soft and golden. Add the cooked lentils, the remaining oil and herbs or spices, mash together and season to taste.

Place the aubergine shells on an oiled oven tray, fill with the mixture and scatter over the topping.

Bake for 30 minutes or until aubergines are soft and the top is golden brown.

Curry, chickpea & squash

stove top

serves 4

Chickpeas are low FODMAP in smaller amounts, so this curry is a good way to benefit from their fibre without over-using them. Make this the night before serving for a richer flavour.

- *450g (1lb) peeled butternut squash, cut into 2cm (¾in) cubes*
- *2 carrots, roughly chopped*
- *2 tbsp oil*
- *2 tbsp of mild curry powder or 2 tsp ground coriander, ground cumin or turmeric, or 3 cardamom pods, or ¼ tsp chilli flakes*
- *1 tbsp green part of spring onions, finely chopped (optional)*
- *350g (12oz) tin of chickpeas, drained and rinsed*
- *1 x 400g tin of coconut milk*
- *1 tbsp finely chopped coriander (cilantro) leaves*
- *salt and pepper*

Steam the squash and carrots in a steamer for about 12 minutes, until just done.

Meanwhile, sauté the spices and spring onion, if using, for 1 minute. Add the carrots and squash, stir, then add the chickpeas and coconut milk. Adjust the flavours to taste, simmer for 10 minutes and stir in the coriander.

Serve with rice and spicy potatoes.

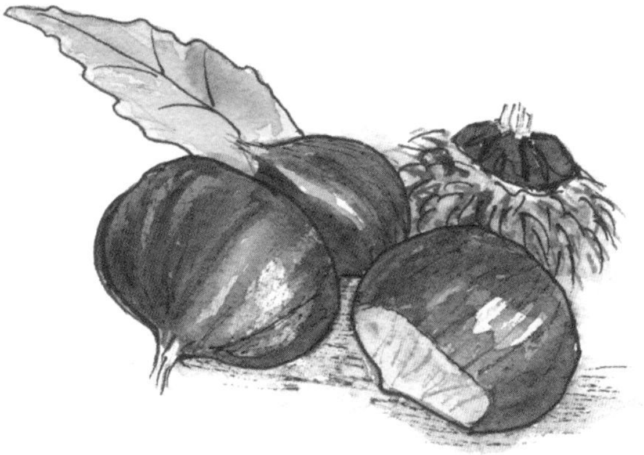

Rice

stove top

serves 4

Every curry needs a good rice dish and this is very good. Rice is a staple for people following a FODMAP diet. Allow 50–75g (2–3oz) of rice per person depending on whether it's being served as a side dish or main

- *1 tbsp green part of spring onion, finely chopped*
- *1 tbsp oil for frying*
- *5 cardamom seeds*
- *2–3 cloves*
- *1 tsp fennel seeds*
- *1 tsp onion seeds (nigella)*
- *200–300g (8–12oz) basmati rice, rinsed*

In a pan which has a closely fitting lid, sauté the onion until soft. Add the spices, fry for 1 minute, then add the rice and fry for 1 minute.

Remove from heat and pour enough water over the rice so that it is double the volume, clap on the lid, reduce the heat to the lowest setting and simmer for 16 minutes.

Take off the heat, replace the lid with a clean tea towel and stand the pan in a warm place until ready to serve.

Chestnut stuffing

serves 4

Although chestnuts can be high FODMAP in quantities of over 165g (6oz) per person, this stuffing is way below that. It also packs a lot of flavour. This stuffing can be used as a filling for pastry rolls or for stuffing chicken or marrow.

- *200g (7oz) cooked and peeled chestnuts*
- *1 tbsp herbs – rosemary, sage or thyme*
- *1 tbsp oil + 1 tsp for oiling tray if using*
- *1 small onion, grated (optional)*
- *1 garlic clove, chopped (optional)*
- *salt and pepper*

Combine all the ingredients in a bowl ready for use.

Bake the stuffing in an oiled tray for 20 minutes or add extra 20 minutes cooking time, if you are stuffing a roast.

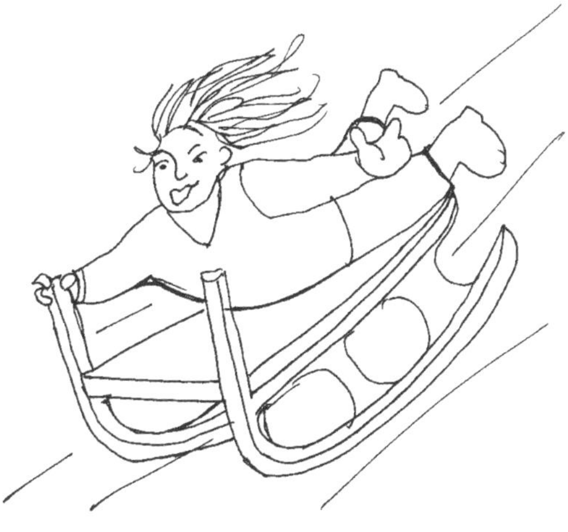

I recently catered for a family on the GAPS diet and the mother started crying. I asked why and she said they were tears of gratitude as no-one had ever cooked a GAPS meal for them before.

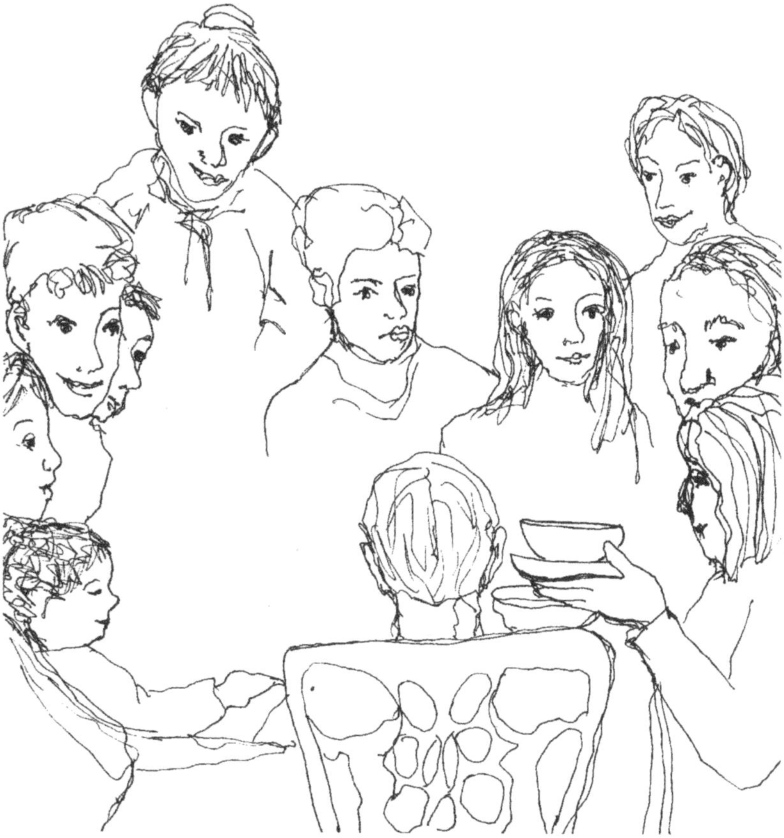

GAPS DIET

The Gut and Psychology Syndrome diet (GAPS) is a variant of SCD (specific carbohydrate diet), although it is more restrictive.

SCD limits the use of complex carbohydrates (disaccharides and polysaccharides). The only carbs you are allowed to eat while you are on the SCD are those that are the least effort to digest and are gentle on the intestines. SCD was designed to help combat gastrointestinal disorders like IBS, ulcerative colitis, Crohn's disease, coeliac disease and inflammatory bowel disease. Monosaccharides are allowed and various foods including fish, aged cheese and honey are included. Prohibited foods include cereal grains, potatoes and lactose-containing dairy products.

Mary

Mary always had health problems. A glandular fever-type illness when she was in her mid-teens led to her taking lots of antibiotic medicine. She felt bloated, ill and depressed as a young adult.

She went on the GAPS diet and, after starting the introductory part, where she felt much better, she experienced huge amounts of bloating after eating a bowl of butternut squash soup.

She took several tests which showed she had fructose malabsorption and that she was not producing hydrochloric acid in her stomach. Now she takes digestive enzymes for the hydrochloric acid. She says, 'My advice is to record what you're eating and your subsequent symptoms. If you have experienced dysbiosis for years, you may need to undergo various tests to determine what underlying issues you need to address before starting on the GAPS diet.'

She is no longer on the GAPS diet, has no stomach pain or abdominal symptoms and is happy and healthy.

Misha

Misha lasted two weeks on the GAPS diet as she found it too difficult to source ingredients in her very rural area. However, during the diet, she found her normally over-quick mind cleared and became slower than it had been for years. She occasionally goes back to the diet when she feels the need to slow down.

The GAPS diet utilises many of the same restrictions as SCD but is structured differently and further restricts carbohydrate intake.

The whole idea behind the GAPS diet is that by eating certain foods you can improve both your digestion and your psychological and emotional health. It is believed that a variety of conditions are caused by an intestinal issue known as leaky gut (aka increased intestinal permeability), and that leaky gut syndrome can lead to psychological and emotional issues as the immune system tries to respond to released toxins.

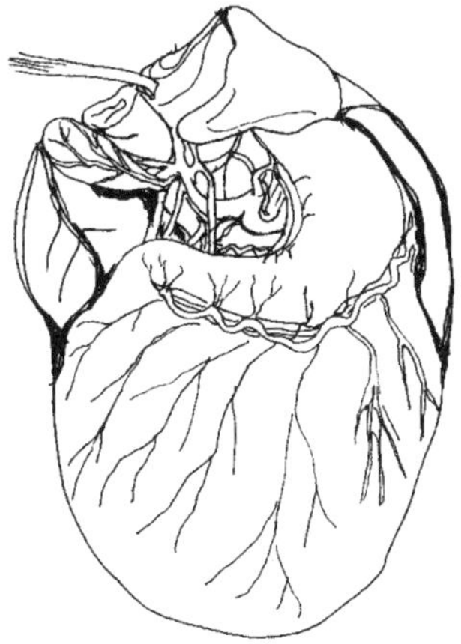

Gastrointestinal perforations can occur due to diverticulitis and other ailments. The omentum (*right*) – a large apron-like expanse of fatty tissue that encases the liver, intestine and stomach and which contains growth factors and elements – adheres to and mends these holes. The omentum also plays a part in the immune system but its role is only now being discovered.

The GAPS diet is designed to last only a couple of years, with the hope that once it is over, the patient will have fully recovered and will be able to resume normal eating patterns.

Like SCD, GAPS is a controversial diet and by no means all nutritionists, doctors and mainstream scientists believe in its efficacy – and some are completely dismissive of it. Those who do believe in it say that word of mouth and online testimonials speak for themselves.

The GAPS diet is only part of what is called 'The Nutritional Protocol'. This is broken into three parts, specifically designed to heal and seal the gut lining, rebalance the immune system and restore the optimal bacterial biome within the gastro-intestinal tract.
The Nutritional Protocol combines the diet, supplements (because of restrictions in the diet there is a need for multi-vitamins and mineral supplements) and detoxification.

If you are cooking for someone on the GAPS diet it is important to work in collaboration with them, even if it is only for one meal, as the foods they can eat change over the course of the two years.

Typical foods allowed

- **fresh meat, preferably hormone-free and grass-fed**
- **animal fats, such as lard, tallow, lamb fat, duck fat, raw butter and ghee**
- **fish**
- **shellfish**
- **organic eggs**
- **fermented foods, such as kefir, homemade yogurt and sauerkraut**
- **vegetables**

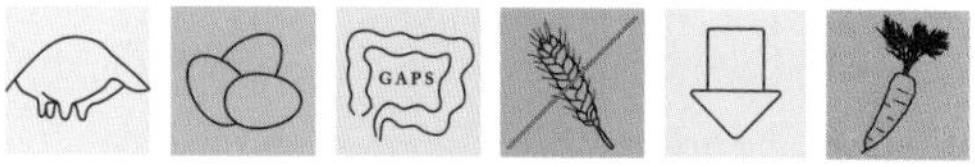

Carrot & courgette bake

moderate oven

serves 4

Serve this instead of a quiche or pie to your friends on a GAPS diet.

You can make a lighter version by beating the egg whites separately before adding them to the mix.

- *25g (1oz) sesame seeds (optional)*
- *3 small carrots, grated*
- *3 small courgettes (zucchini), grated*
- *1 small onion, finely chopped*
- *1 garlic clove, minced*
- *1 tbsp oil, for frying and a little for greasing*
- *4 eggs, beaten*
- *100g (4oz) grated Cheddar cheese, feta or manchego*
- *1 tsp dried mixed herbs*
- *salt and pepper*

Heat the oven to 180°C/ fan160°C/350°F/Gas 4.

Toast the seeds in a dry frying pan for a minute or so until toasted and fragrant. Tip out into a bowl and set to one side.

Sauté the vegetables and garlic in the pan with the oil until just soft, then transfer to a bowl and allow to cool. Add the seeds, beaten eggs, cheese, herbs and seasoning. Place in a greased, deep baking dish and bake in the oven for 20–30 minutes until golden and firm.

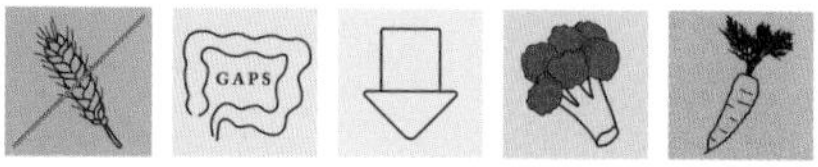

Cauliflower mash

stove top

per person

There are many cauliflower GAP recipes and lots of them start with this mash. Use this mash as a substitute for potato on fish pie or Anglesey eggs (page 22).

- *75g (3oz) cauliflower*
- *1 tsp salad oil or butter*
- *salt and pepper*

Split the cauliflower into florets and steam for about 10 minutes until soft. Drain really well in a colander, then return to the pan and mash with oil or butter and season.

If you like, try toasting the mash in a dry frying pan for a few minutes, just before serving.

Mind the GAP

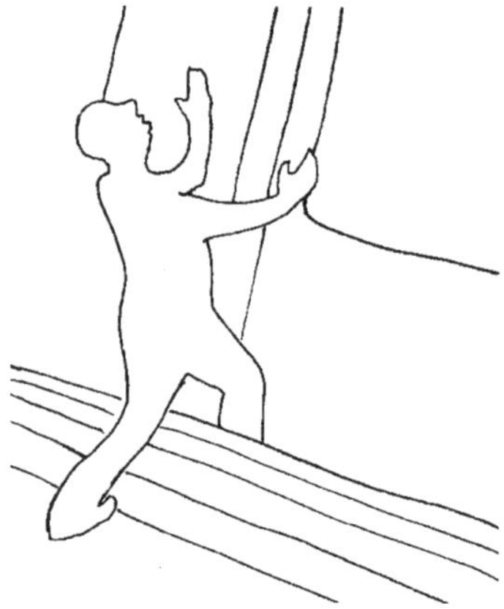

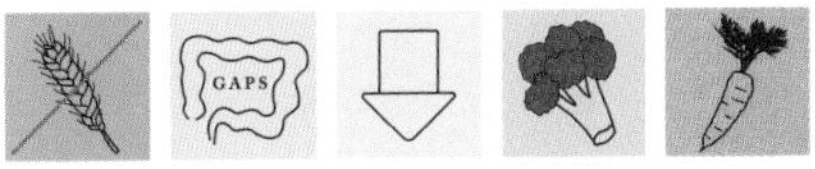

Dahl

stove top

serves 4

Make sure to wash the lentils well. GAPS experts suggest that you wash and drain, simmer and stir as the best way to cook lentils and of course always from fresh as in this recipe. Dahl can be as thick as hummus to stuff into pitta bread or as thin as cream to serve with curries. Try adding a handful of chopped spinach leaves and 1 tablespoon of chopped coriander (cilantro).

per person

- *110g (4oz) red lentils, washed*
- *1 tsp salt*
- *3 bay leaves*
- *200ml (7fl oz) cold water*
- *1 tbsp creamed coconut*
- *2 tsp curry powder or ½ tsp ground coriander, 1 tsp ground cumin, 1 tsp ground turmeric, 2 whole cloves*

Put the washed lentils, salt and bay leaves in a pan with the cold water and bring to the boil. Simmer until the lentils are very soft, adding more water if they become dry.

In a cup, soften the coconut with 1 tablespoon of boiling water and stir into the lentils. Add the spices and cook everything for a further 5 minutes.

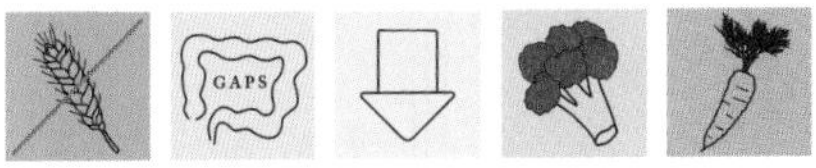

Garlic & ginger carrots

stove top

serves 4

Anti-inflammatory ginger and garlic may sound medicinal, but this dish is just gorgeously spicy.

- *3 medium carrots, cut into 5cm (2in) x 1cm (3/8in) lengths*
- *1 tbsp oil*
- *1 tbsp grated fresh root ginger*
- *2 cloves minced garlic*
- *1 tsp honey or maple syrup*
- *salt and pepper*

Fry the carrots and ginger over a low heat in a pan with the lid on, stirring often, for 15 minutes, then add the garlic and stir well, replacing lid for further 5 minutes.

Stir through the honey or maple syrup to coat all the carrots before serving.

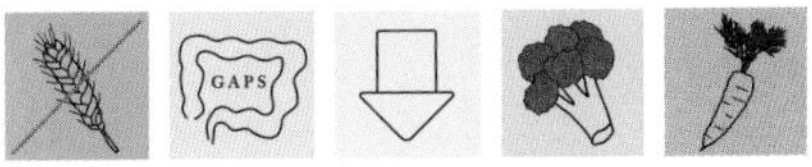

Gremolata

serves 4

A GAPS favourite to brighten and flavour plain dishes or to eat as an accompaniment to fish, meat or vegetables. Serve on baked aubergine, grilled meats or fish.

- *3 tbsp chopped parsley*
- *2 medium garlic cloves*
- *grated zest of ½ lemon, plus juice (optional)*
- *salt and pepper*

Finely chop the parsley and garlic together and transfer to a small bowl. Add the zest and chop through again, then add the lemon juice, if using. Season to taste.

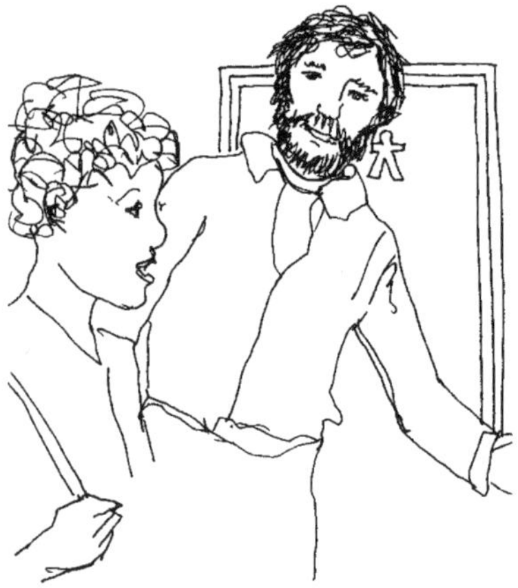

I feel a little more human now.

I feel that's a little too much information!

Right: Fitting within the skin: Your chest cavity holds the lungs and heart. Your liver and spleen sit just below the ribs and your squashy belly in front of the hips and spine is home to the large intestine, which looks here like lots of sausages on a string, is home to the millions of friends we share our body with.

GUT BIOME & IBD

Inside each of us is a beautiful little paradise. Here, minute beings live out their entire lives and we benefit from some and are harmed by others, as they produce their various by-products and wastes. These beings are the gut flora and the paradise is the gut biome.

The gut biome is an ecosystem made up of all the bacteria and other microbes that colonise our gastrointestinal tract. It is not static and it changes throughout life, after the first colonisation at birth. Variation is highest during childhood and it gradually decreases with age. Illness, antibiotic use, fever, stress, injury and dietary changes all affect the blend of microbes that make up the biome.

Science suggests that the disorder of our microbial ecology may well be a major contributor to the modern epidemics of allergy, autoimmune disease, obesity and diabetes. Lower bacterial diversity has been observed in people with diseases such as inflammatory bowel disease, psoriatic arthritis, type 1 and type 2 diabetes, atopic eczema, coeliac disease and obesity. The association between reduced diversity and disease indicates that a species-rich gut biome is more robust against environmental influences.

Lily

Poor little baby Lily, great red patches blistered and scabbed her face. She seemed to have impetigo, which is unusual in a four-month-old child. Two courses of antibiotics failed to clear it up and added to her misery and that of her parents. Firstly, they had to force the medicine into her mouth as she fought them and screamed, and then she had extreme diarrhoea, which woke them all up every night. It was a terrible month until her mum realised from researching online that what Lily had was not impetigo but an uncommon form of eczema.

This breastfed baby and her mum began an elimination diet. First to go were acids, then cereals and cereal flours – wheat especially. Next were cow's milk, cheese and butter.

Gradually her face symptoms began to clear up and it seems now that it isn't just one food or food group that causes those great red welts to suddenly reappear, rather it is combination and abundance. If Lily has too many nuts or seeds the skin of her body becomes lumpy and rough. She avoids commercial crisps cooked in sunflower oil, her mum substitutes rapeseed oil for sunflower and makes her own crisps.

Lily's diet contains a lot of dark bone broth – and she still loves it, as well as goat's cheese, avocado, spelt bread and buckwheat pancakes.

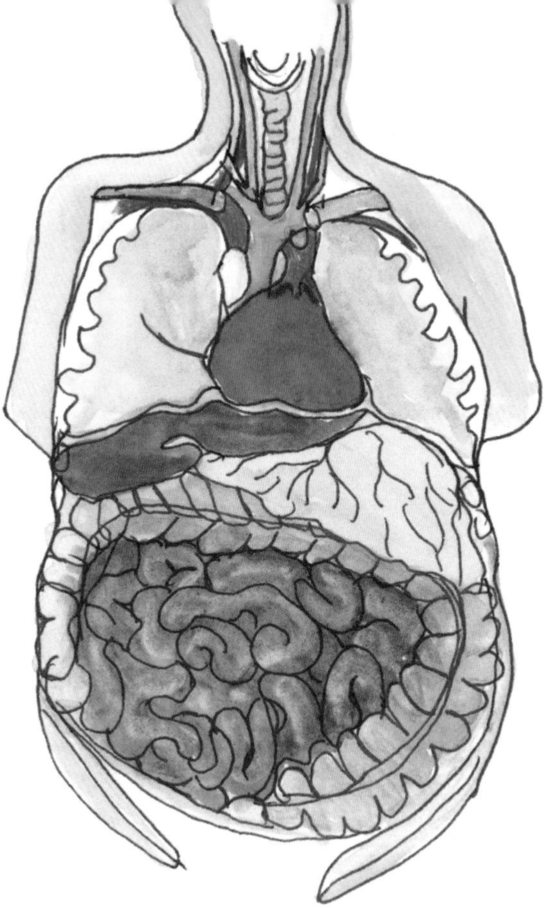

Many chronic conditions can be mitigated against, though not necessarily cured, by adjusting the nutrients available to the beneficial bacteria in our gut. This enables them to flourish and provide us with all we need to thrive. When the gut biome is balanced we feel well, healthy and alert. But when it goes wrong, whether acutely or chronically, we suffer.

Over 300,000 people in the UK live with long-term inflammatory bowel conditions that result in symptoms like chronic diarrhoea, which can lead to 20–30 trips to the loo daily.

The stress of living with the consequences of any bowel ailment also affects the gut. Stress is detrimental to the gut flora, because adrenalin prioritises blood flow to muscles and nerves and away from the gut. This leads to dysbiosis, which is pro-inflammatory and aggravates the gut lining, leading to food intolerance and autoimmune disease. This can, in turn, deplete certain nutrients such as magnesium and B vitamins. All of which leads to a vicious cycle of stress and further loss of microbiome diversity and uncomfortable abdominal symptoms.

Emil

Emil inherited what he calls a compromised digestion. He was raised as a vegetarian though the family sometimes ate fish.

When he was in India in 2018 he suffered a bout of typhoid and had to have 10 days of strong antibiotics, which left him with exhaustion. Afterwards he ate a simple diet of rice, yogurt, papaya and egg and seemed fine, though the symptoms of low energy continued.

Last year after eating a croissant he had gas, bloating and such sharp pain that he had to lie down. He eventually burped painfully and his symptoms then went away. All the symptoms came back after every meal, though, no matter what he ate.

He researched SIBO (small intestine bacterial overload diet, a bit like FODMAP). Emil found eating only small meals helped but left him tired. Then, 10 days later, his mother recommended that he see a Chinese herbalist who was also an acupuncturist.

The herbalist took his pulse and looked at his tongue and said he had chronically bad digestion which was extreme for his age. He had some acupuncture treatment, some instructions to eat very few carbs, no cold beverages, no pulses, sugar or raw food and to increase his protein intake. He was given what the herbalist called, herbs for quiet digestion and says that, though he didn't know what they were, he felt better straight away. All the symptoms faded after a time, though whenever he ran out of herbs, they would reappear.

Emil stayed on the diet and felt better overall. Two months later the herbalist gave him The Six Gentlemen (ginseng, liquorice, atractylodes, poria, citrus peel and pinellia root), to build up strength in his digestion. He has continued with the diet and eats almost no raw food or pulses, and more fish for the protein.

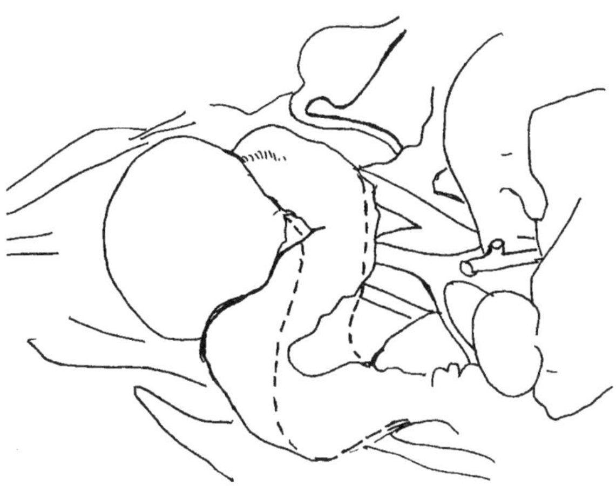

When lying down, the full colon is displaced

IBD & Crohn's disease

People with bowel disease not only have to put up with the symptoms of their illness but also suffer from the prejudice of other people. For instance, 52 per cent of people in the UK with Crohn's disease said they have experienced discrimination because of their condition.

IBD, or inflammatory bowel disease, is a term mainly used to describe two conditions: ulcerative colitis and Crohn's disease. These are long-term conditions that involve inflammation of the gut.

Ulcerative colitis only affects the colon (large intestine), but Crohn's disease can affect any part of the digestive system. While the causes of Crohn's disease are unknown, it seems to be due to a combination of environmental, immune and bacterial factors in genetically susceptible individuals. It results in a chronic inflammatory disorder, in which the body's immune system attacks the gastrointestinal tract.

People of any age can have IBD, but it's usually diagnosed between the ages of 15 and 40. Rates of IBD have been increasing, particularly in the developing world, since the 1970s and currently there is no cure for ulcerative colitis or Crohn's disease.

Certain foods and beverages can aggravate the symptoms of IBD, especially during a flare-up. As a result, many people with this condition find that problems such as diarrhoea, abdominal pain and gas improve by limiting or eliminating dairy products, saturated-fat foods and limiting high-fibre foods such as fresh fruits, raw vegetables and whole grains. They choose instead foods which are steamed, baked or stewed.

People with Crohn's disease of the small intestine may not be able to digest or absorb fat normally. Instead, fat passes quickly along the intestine, making diarrhoea worse. Thus, they avoid butter, margarine, cream sauces and fried foods. In general, they may also have more problems with foods in the cabbage family, nuts, seeds, corn and popcorn. Spicy foods, alcohol and caffeine may also make symptoms worse.

People with IBD are recommended to eat small meals and drink plenty of liquids.

Diverticulosis

Diverticula are small, bulging pouches that can form in the lining of the colon or large intestine creating a condition called diverticulosis. In some cases, one or more diverticula can become inflamed or infected, which is called diverticulitis.

People with diverticulosis, a common condition among older people, usually adopt a high-fibre diet which includes vegetables, fruit, nuts, seeds, legumes (beans, split peas and lentils), brown rice, wholegrain breads and cereals. But if they have a flare up of diverticulitis, they may be reduced to eating only broth and fruit juices, such as apple juice, without pulp. After the acute phase is over, they can slowly add low-fibre foods such as canned or cooked fruits without skin or seeds, canned or cooked vegetables such as green beans, carrots and potatoes (without the skin), eggs, fish and poultry, refined white bread, some cereals, milk, yogurt and cheese, white rice, pasta and noodles, before resuming their normal diet.

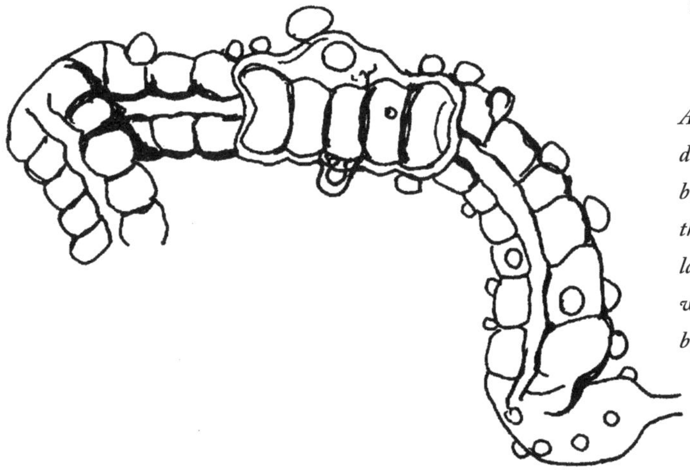

A length of intestine with diverticulosis showing the little bubbles of the diverticular pushing through the muscular wall of the large intestine. Diverticulitis occurs when digested food within the bubbles become infected.

Joseph

Joseph always ate a diet with lots of vegetables and wholegrain foods. Five years ago he had symptoms – including traces of blood in his stools and a low-level ache on the left side of his stomach – that led to him being given a colonoscopy. It was obviously a relief not to have bowel cancer, but he was surprised to be diagnosed with diverticulitis, a condition that has symptoms including chronic stomach pain, constipation and diarrhoea.

Apparently 30 per cent of people over 50 in western Europe and the US suffer from this. It seems that the typical patient has over many years eaten a diet of highly refined foods with not enough vegetables or roughage. Another cause may be not drinking enough water and he says that may be a lesson for many people.

After the investigation, Joseph didn't have the usual symptoms most of the time but did suffer unpleasant episodes which included bleeding. About six months after the investigation, he included in his diet lots of tasty and exciting live fermented foods. He started making and enjoying kimchi, kombucha and kefir, as well as lots of lovely organic fresh veg.

He has now been symptom-free since following this diet, as well as enjoying the making, eating and drinking of the foods in his new diet. He is also now enthusiastically brewing live traditional ginger beer, with all its friendly bacteria adding to the range of good things in his gut!

The gut–brain connection or axis

The gut–brain axis transmits information via the vagus nerve from the gut to the brain.

Digested food particles enter the small intestine, which is covered with a velvety layer of hair-like villi – tiny finger-like projections that line the small intestine. Each villus is lined with a single layer of epithelium. This layer is made up of different cell types. One of them, the enteroendocrine cell, is unlike the others. It is our gut sensor and is called a neuropod cell. In addition to communicating through hormones, the neuropod cells also connect with nerves, including the vagus nerve.

Neuropod cells sense and react to their environment. They sense mechanical, thermal and chemical stimuli such as nutrients or bacterial by-products in the gut. In the neuropod cells the signals from stimuli are converted to tiny electrical pulses. These pulses travel via synapses onto the vagus nerve.

Vagal neurons carry the sensory info to the brain stem, linking the signals to the brain. The neuropod connection with the vagus nerve serves as a conduit for food in the gut to influence brain function within seconds, and thoughts and feelings such as stress can be communicated to the gut and affect the gut biome. This connection is also a potential conduit of gut pathogens to access the brain.

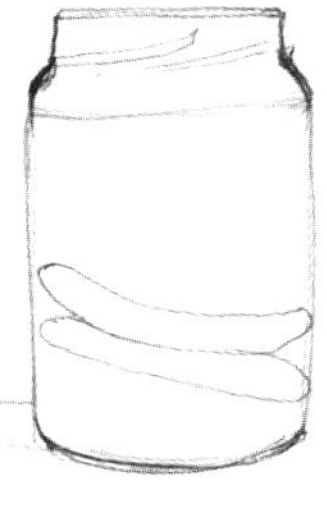

Kombucha: healing the gut, one scobie at a time.

Kimchi

makes 1–2 jars

Kimchi can be quite mild and used as a side dish or it can be made superhot, by adding more ginger and some chilli, when it is best eaten like pickle. Either way it will restore your bacteria and help your digestion long term.

- *1 Chinese cabbage, finely chopped*
- *3 spring onions, finely chopped*
- *1 carrot, grated*
- *1 large white radish, finely chopped*
- *1 tbsp grated fresh root ginger*
- *1 tbsp salt*
- *2 cabbage leaves*

Put all the ingredients in a bowl and strew with the salt. Leave the bowl covered overnight to soften the vegetables. Next morning, with clean hands, press and wring out the veg for about 10 minutes until the juices run.

Pack the veg and the juices tightly into a large clean jar or sauerkraut crock and press firmly down. Lay the whole cabbage leaves over everything and place a clean weight (such as a small, sealed jar of water) on top to keep it all under the juices and the brine.

To make the brine, mix 1 tsp of salt with 500ml (18fl oz) water. Top up with more brine, making sure there is more than two inches of liquid over the weight and the leaves. Place a cloth over the top and set aside on a cool shelf or in the fridge. Do not seal the jar as the gases of fermentation need to escape. Wait for up to 3 weeks before tasting (though it will be fine after 1 week).

Always use a clean spoon to decant the kimchi and always keep the vegetables covered in brine. You can decant into smaller jars to serve and keep in the fridge.

Kombucha

makes 2 bottles

Kombucha has a recorded history as far back as 220 BCE when it helped restore the digestive health of a Chinese emperor. It was probably around for millennia before that. Ask a friend for a scoby, the fruiting body of kombucha, a symbiosis of acetic acid bacteria and osmophilic yeast species. It looks like a brown soft frisbee. Use a 5-litre (1-gallon) glass, heatproof jar with a wide top and a tap – do not use plastic or metal and keep everything scrupulously clean. To close the top, use a fine woven cloth and an elastic band.

- *2 green tea bags*
- *2 black tea bags*
- *150g (5oz) white or coconut sugar*
- *1½ litres (2½ pints) hot water*
- *1 tsp lemon juice or vinegar (optional)*
- *1 scoby*

Make the tea in the jar by pouring boiling water over all the tea bags and stir in the sugar. Steep until cool. Remove the tea bags, then add the Scoby and close the top with the cloth and band.

Leave at room temperature until fermented (around 2 weeks). Use sooner if you like it sweet, later for vinegary taste.

New scobies will appear in the liquid. As the original scoby divides you can give them to a friend or put them on the compost heap.

After syphoning, the kombucha tea can be flavoured with ginger and lemon and refrigerated before serving. Add a new brew of cooled tea to the old scoby to revitalise it. Scobies can live on for years.

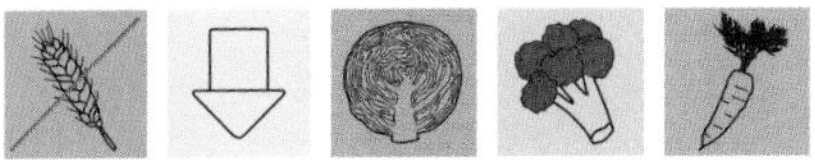

Sauerkraut

makes 1–2 jars

Sauerkraut, along with kimchi, kombucha and Andy's ginger beer (see pages 101, 103), help to readjust the balance of gut microflora. A German friend says we use sauerkraut too young and it is best after 6 months!

- *1 medium cabbage, finely chopped, but save a couple of outside leaves*
- *salt (2% to weight of cabbage – a 500g cabbage would need 10g/¼oz of salt)*
- *1 tbsp caraway seed*

Brine

- *1 tsp of salt mixed with 500ml (18fl oz) water*

Put the cabbage in a bowl, strew with the salt and leave it covered overnight to soften.

Next day, with clean hands, press and wring it for about 10 minutes until it releases its juice. Stir in the caraway seed. Pack it down tightly and firmly into a large clean jar or sauerkraut crock with the juices. Lay the reserved leaves over the veg and place the weight on top to keep it all under the briny juice. Top up with more brine, if necessary, until there is more than 8cm (3in) over the weight and leaves. Place a clean cloth over the top and set aside at room temperature. Wait for up to 3 weeks before tasting, checking every few days if the brine needs a top up.

If scum forms on the top of the liquid, spoon it away and top up with fresh brine.

Always use a clean spoon to decant the sauerkraut and keep it covered in brine.

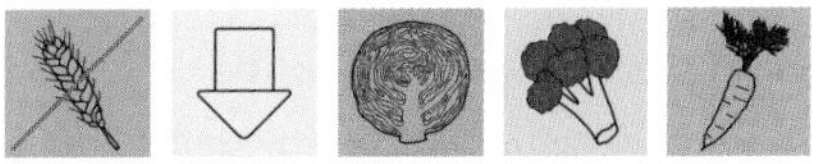

Olive tapenade

serves 4

Olives are a good source of dietary fibre for good gut health and are also rich in iron and copper. Eating olives and using olive oil are said to enhance your life expectancy. A good substitute for anchovies in recipes and on pizzas. For a less salty taste, wash the olives first.

- *100g (3½oz) pitted olives (watch out for citric acid and colouring)*
- *3 tbsp extra virgin olive oil*
- *2 garlic cloves, finely chopped*
- *2 tbsp chopped parsley*

Put all the ingredients in a blender and whiz until it becomes a thick paste. Add more oil if it's too thick.

When you're feeling sour,
All a-pickle and a-pout,
Fetch yourself a cabbage
And make some Sauerkraut.

Diolch, Wil a Lois
(thank you, Wil and Lois)

Meat broth

stove top

makes 1–2 jars

Meat broth is especially good for people with IBD to help mend the intestinal walls. Essentially providing the building blocks for rapid healthy growth of intestinal lining cells.

- *450g (1lb) raw bones of organic lamb, chicken or beef*
- *salt and pepper (optional)*

Boil the bones in a pan of water for about 4 hours or until any flesh on them drops away. Cool and then strain the broth.

Transfer to a clean jar with a lid, store in a fridge and drink a cupful a day. Or you can pour it into small containers and batch-freeze it to use as a base for gravies, soups and stews.

Hedgerow broth

stove top

makes 1–2 jars

For everyone who does not eat meat, this broth can help regrowth of a healthy gut biome and restore the intestinal lining cells after they have been affected by IBD. It's also very tasty and full of vitamins, minerals and antioxidants.

- *450g (1lb) mix of washed hedgerow fruits – sloes, haws, rosehips, blackberries, crab apples*

Combine all the ingredients in a pan and simmer together until all the fruits are soft.

Cool and strain the broth through a sieve lined with a fine-weave cloth (especially if using rosehips).

Transfer to a jar with a lid and store in the fridge, or batch-freeze in small amounts to use as a base for gravies, soups and stews.

Fried bananas

stove top

per person

Often cited as one of the superfoods your gut needs, bananas can be boring but not like this. Serve up to unexpected dinner guests knowing that their gut biome will love them. If you're serving these to adults, add 1 tablespoon of brandy to the pan at the last moment for a flambéed treat.

- *1 banana, sliced lengthways or across*
- *1 tsp coconut oil or butter*

On a low heat, fry the banana in a frying pan in the coconut oil or butter until golden brown on both sides.

Serve alone or with ice-cream.

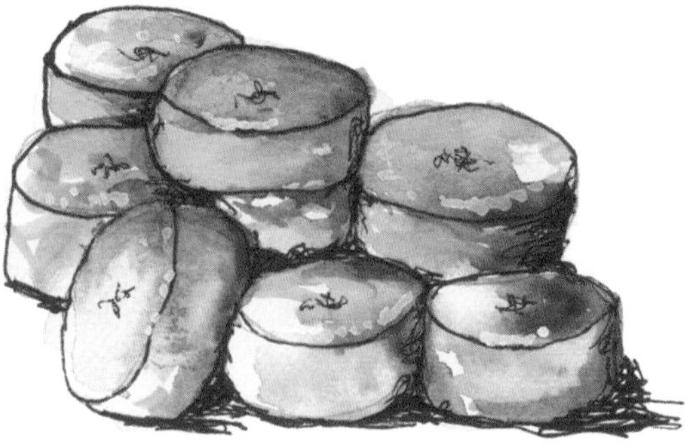

Andy's ginger beer (a long-term project)

makes 6 litres (10 pints)

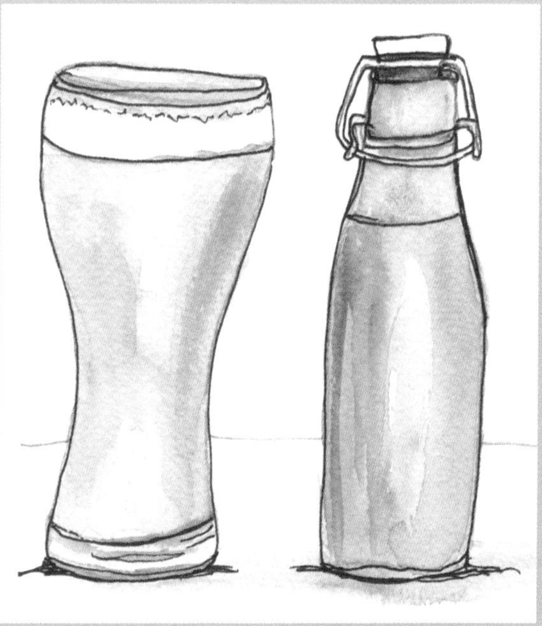

Ginger beer is a long-term project or a lifetime habit. Andy, who gave me this recipe, swears it has improved his gut health and wellbeing hugely.

Do not use metal equipment.

- *500ml (18fl oz) filtered water*
- *8 raisins*
- *juice of 2 lemons*
- *8 x 8 tbsp finely grated ginger*
- *8 x 8 tbsp sugar*
- *6–8 tbsp sugar*
- *1 litre (1¾ pints) boiling water, plus 1 litre (1¾ pints) of cold*
- *juice of 3 lemons*
- *5 litres (1 gallon) cold water*

In a large jar, mix the water, raisins and lemon juice with 1 tablespoon of ginger and 1 tablespoon of sugar, cover with a cloth and secure with a rubber band.

Feed this for a week by adding 1 tablespoon of ginger and 1 tablespoon of sugar daily. After a few days it should start bubbling and fizzing when you add the sugar.

If nothing is happening after 8 days, throw it away and start again.

Now you should be ready to start the beer. In a large heatproof basin, dissolve the sugar in the boiling water, stirring, then add the 1 litre (1¾ pints) cold water.

Into a 5-litre (1-gallon) container, strain and squeeze the juice from the plant mixture, reserving the plant. Add 3 litres (5 pints) cold water and the lemon juice to the plant juice.

Keep the plant and feed it every day as before or store it in the fridge to revive later.

When the sugar water is at body temperature or cooler, add it to the container and stir well.

Transfer to clean plastic or flip-top beer bottles, leaving a gap of 5cm (2in) at the neck.

Keep in a warm place and open the bottles after 3 days to release some of the built-up gas. Do this every day to prevent the bottles from popping.

The beer will be ready to drink in one week or a little longer if the air temperature is cooler.

They smell delicious but the hole in the doughnut is the only part I can eat!

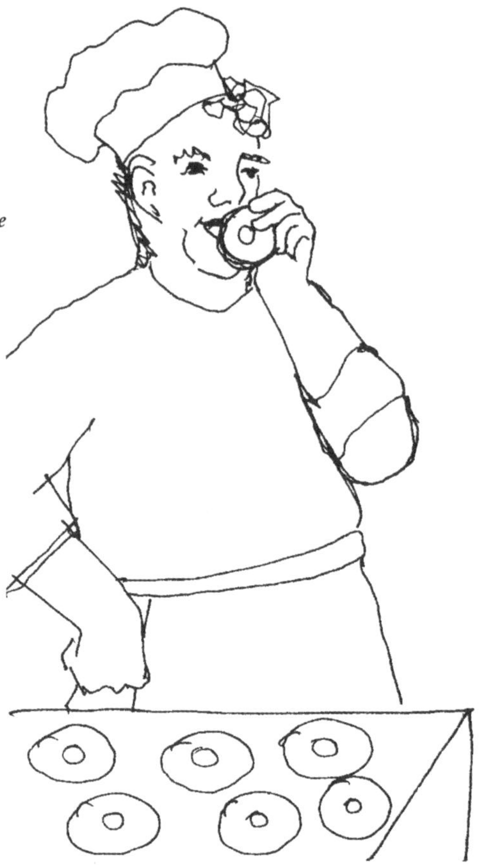

IBS & FIBRE

Irritable Bowel Syndrome

IBS is a term that encompasses a group of symptoms including abdominal pain and changes in the pattern of bowel movements without any evidence of underlying damage. In medical terms IBS is defined by the presence of recurrent abdominal pain associated with disordered defecation in the absence of demonstrable organic disease. In lay terms this means you have painful bloating and wind, and bouts of diarrhoea and constipation but there is no disease present.

The condition affects 10–15 per cent of the population but it is thought that only 10–25 per cent of people who suffer from IBS seek medical care.

The causes of IBS are not clear, though it is thought to be a gut motor-sensory disorder, the basis of which may be physiological, but it is affected by various environmental factors such as certain foods and other elements such as stress, illness and psychological or physiological problems. It can be associated with weight loss, colitis and inflammatory bowel disease.

Dietary changes are often helpful, so people with IBS are recommended to increase their fibre intake, use probiotics, go on a gluten-free diet or use a FODMAP diet for a short time.

Fibre

Dietary fibre describes plant-based carbohydrates that, unlike sugars and starch, are not digested in the small intestine but reach the large intestine or colon. These include pectin and beta-glucans, found in foods like fruit and oats, and cellulose, found in whole grains and nuts.

A recent study in New Zealand looked at clinical trials which showed there is significantly lower bodyweight, systolic blood pressure and total cholesterol in people with a higher rather than lower intake of dietary fibre. Daily intake of dietary fibre of between 25g and 29g or higher appeared to protect against cardiovascular diseases, type 2 diabetes and colorectal and breast cancers. Similar findings for whole-grain intake were observed.

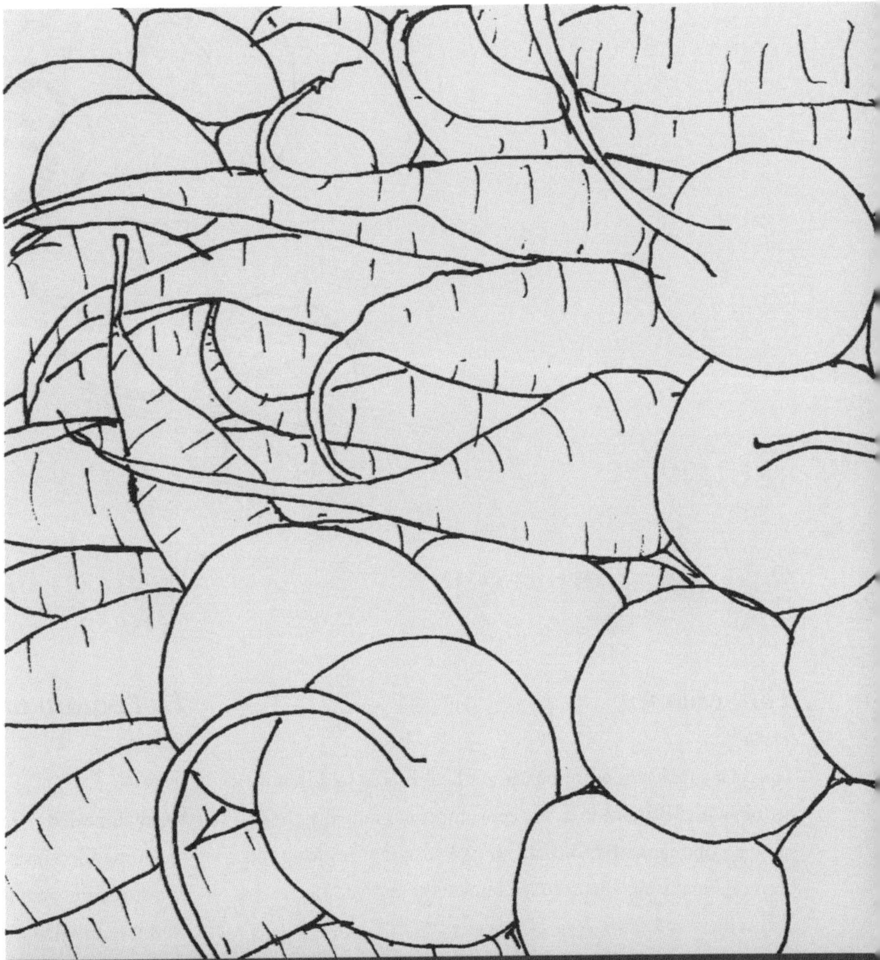

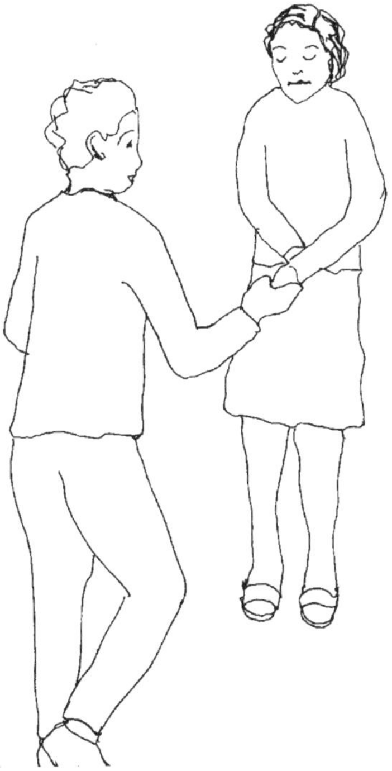

High fibre vegetables are good for many people with IBS but in others can trigger bouts of bloating.

Fibre-rich foods include:

- wholegrain breakfast cereals
- wholewheat pasta
- wholegrain bread
- oats
- barley
- rye
- fruit (berries, pears, melon)
- vegetables (broccoli, carrots, sweetcorn)
- pulses
- nuts and seeds

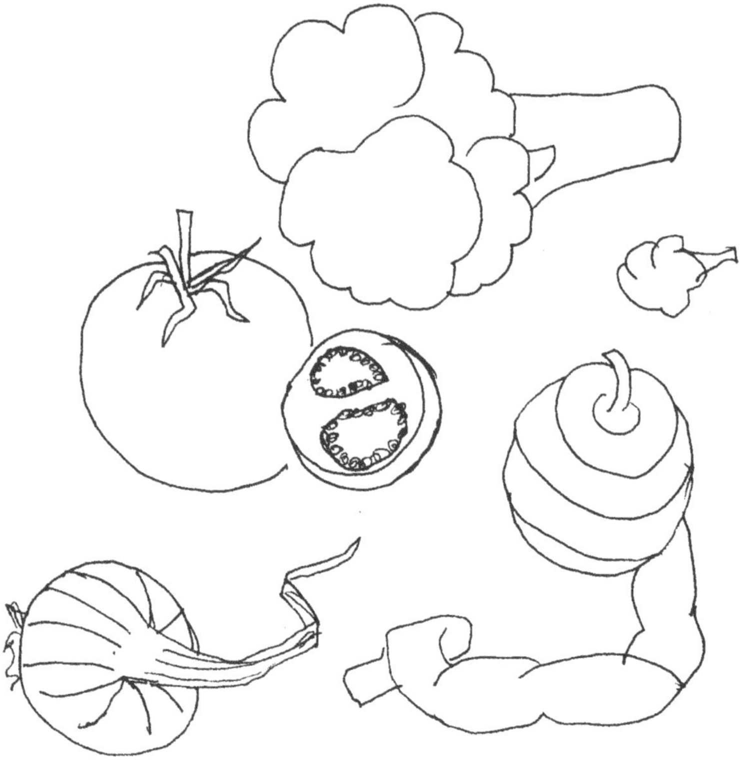

Tofu cream

serves 4

Tofu is a gateway food to better gut health: it is said that if people with IBS ease into soy consumption gradually, the same components that initially provoked symptoms can become beneficial. This tofu cream is light and you need only a little as a sauce over a dessert.

- *225g (8oz) plain silken tofu*
- *½ tsp vanilla extract or ½ vanilla pod*
- *2 tbsp maple or agave syrup*
- *1 tbsp sunflower oil*
- *milk substitute to thin*

Whiz all the ingredients together in a blender to form a smooth cream. This can be as thick as double cream or as thin as milk – whatever you prefer.

Hot potato salad

stove top

serves 4

Waxy unpeeled potatoes are featured in recipes recommended for people with IBS as they are high in fibre and for many people they are not irritating to the gut. For a cold potato salad, cool the potatoes for longer and substitute 2 tablespoons of mayonnaise, or Avocado & sunflower seed mayo dip (page 48), for the oil.

- *450g (1lb) small unpeeled waxy potatoes*
- *2 tbsp olive oil*
- *2 tbsp finely chopped herbs – rosemary, marjoram, mint (optional)*
- *salt and pepper*

Boil the potatoes until just soft and rinse in cold water and cool for 5 minutes. Add the olive oil, herbs, if using, and seasoning. Mix everything together, being careful not to break the potato skins.

Serve immediately.

Thai healing soup

stove top

serves 4

Quick to make and packed with nutrition this soup is also low FODMAP and easy on the digestive system. Ginger is soothing and the vegetables are cooked so quickly they lose few if any of their nutrients.

- *1 x 400g tin of coconut milk*
- *400ml (14fl oz) vegetable stock*
- *1–2 tbsp soy or fish sauce*
- *1 tbsp powdered seaweed (optional)*
- *1 tbsp grated fresh root ginger*
- *3 garlic cloves, minced*
- *1 small red chilli, chopped*
- *pinch of five spice (optional)*
- *2 carrots, thinly cut*
- *½ courgette (zucchini), thinly cut*
- *4 mushrooms, thinly cut*
- *3 spring onions, cut into thin strips*
- *1 red pepper, deseeded and chopped*
- *3 heads of pak choi, chopped longways*
- *2 tbsp chopped basil leaves*
- *1 tbsp chopped coriander (cilantro)*
- *salt and pepper*

In a large pan, simmer together the milk, stock, soy or fish sauce, ginger, garlic, chilli and five spice. Add all the vegetables except the pak choi and herbs, and simmer for 5 minutes.

Add the pak choi, basil, coriander and seasoning. Simmer for 2 minutes.

Serve hot with noodles or sushi rice.

Frozen banana ice

freezer

per person

Bananas are a healer for the gut and can be soothing to people with IBS. Try these with a little tofu cream.

These make excellent lollies if you place them on a stick before freezing.

- *1 banana, peeled*

Chop the bananas in half and place on a tray to batch-freeze. When frozen, they can be bagged up.

Blend to use as ice-cream or as a base for smoothies.

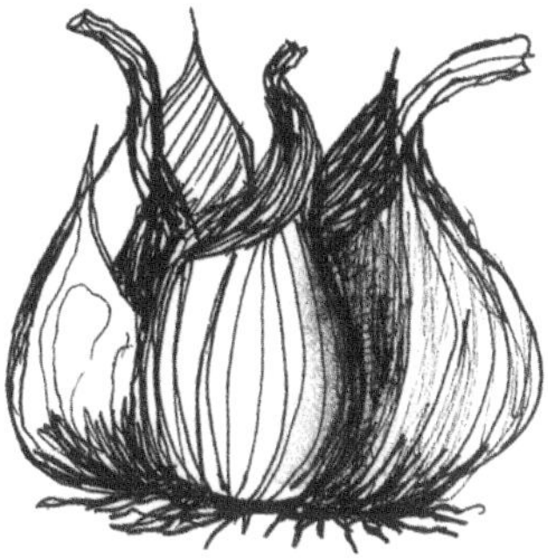

Garlic can be problematic for some people with IBS as it contains fructans (a FODMAP sugar) but for others it is a real help.

ETHICAL EATERS

We are used to people eating different foods for cultural or religious reasons and would always ask for their preferences when making a meal for them. But now there is an awareness of ethical considerations around ingredients, too. Many vegetarians and vegans have chosen their diets for ethical reasons; but there are also other forms of ethical eaters.

In recent years there has been mounting pressure to rethink what we eat in order to reduce carbon consumption. However, cutting our carbon consumption can be complicated.

Lamb from large-scale farming costs up to 5kg / CO_2e (carbon dioxide equivalent) while it is estimated that cashews cost 4.9kg / CO_2e, mangoes 4.4kg / CO_2e, avocados 2.2kg / CO_2e and almonds 2.6kg / CO_2e, when taking into account the amount of waste, special storage and packaging that is needed for them.

Substituting seasonal foods for ones that are available all year, and not flown in from a distance, cuts down on their carbon footprint. This could mean eating hazelnuts from Essex rather than Californian almonds or using pears instead of mangoes in fruit salad.

Locavores (people who eat only locally produced food) would like everyone to reduce the distance their food travels from farm to fork. They say that large-scale meat farms are harmful to the environment because the animals are fed on imported fodder and their meat is shipped great distances. To reduce CO_2 if you are a meat eater, it is better to buy from a local farm where animals have been almost entirely grass-fed.

Let's eat organic food – or food, as our grandparents called it.

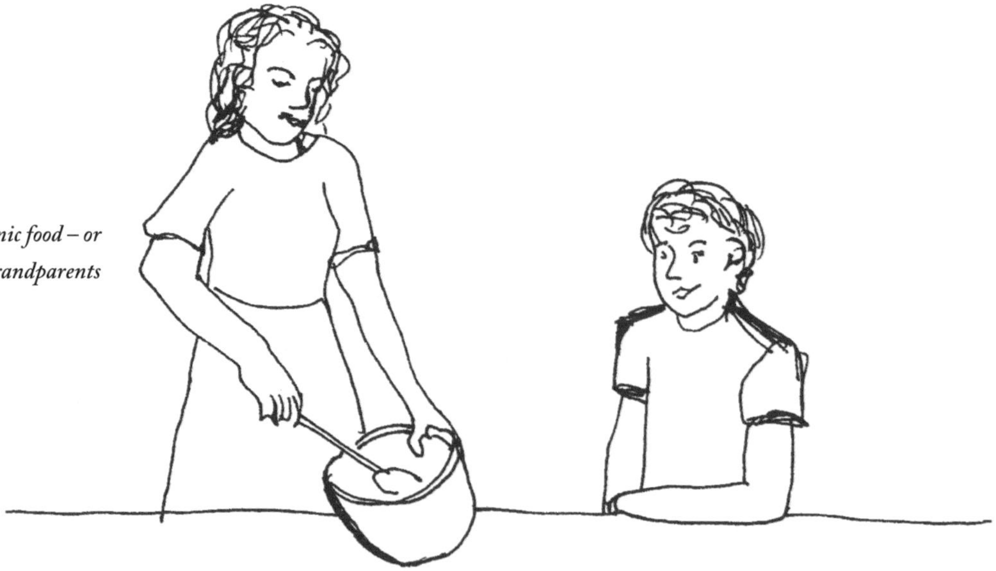

Make your own compost and grow organic vegetables and fruit. Gathering and storing fruit was part of life before industrialisation and fashion robbed us of skills and habits.

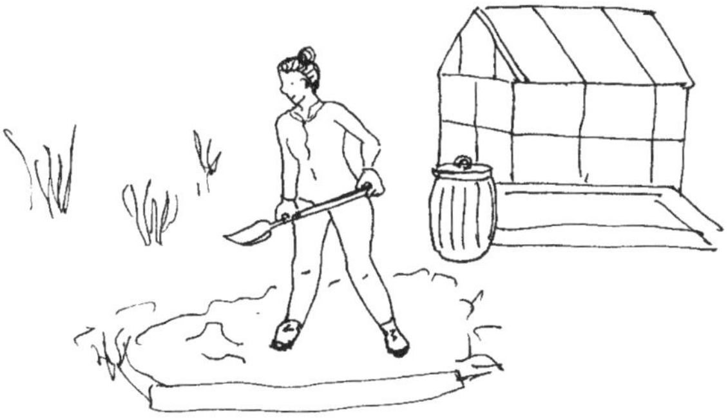

Organic food

In the UK, the Soil Association organic label comes with a host of givens. On organic meat farms the animals are well cared for, the people who rear the animals are themselves well looked after and in turn make sure that the source of the animals' food and what becomes of their waste is all recorded and accounted for. There is an assurance that you will eat a plant or animal that has not been too heavily affected by chemicals and has been picked and processed by someone who has been well respected and given adequate compensation for their work. Not only that but all the stuff around growing and processing has also been considered – from the packaging and advertising all the way back to the air, soil and water. Sometimes the food tastes better, too.

A myth about organic food production is that yields are lower, but many studies have shown that the opposite is the case. Because organic methods of farming build up soil structure and fertility, the resulting yields are comparative, if not better.

Of course, all this care does make the product more expensive to buy, but if you can afford it, buying organic can be one of the first steps to take towards a more accountable and considered approach to buying food. One loaf of bread, a chicken or some apples is not only better for you, but it sends a message out to the food producers that this is what we want. When enough of us ask for organics then the big players will give us just that. After all, they are in business to make money, and if organics and ethical production is where the money is then they will follow. Buying organic whenever you can helps the wheel to turn little by little in the direction of food that is better for us and for the Earth too.

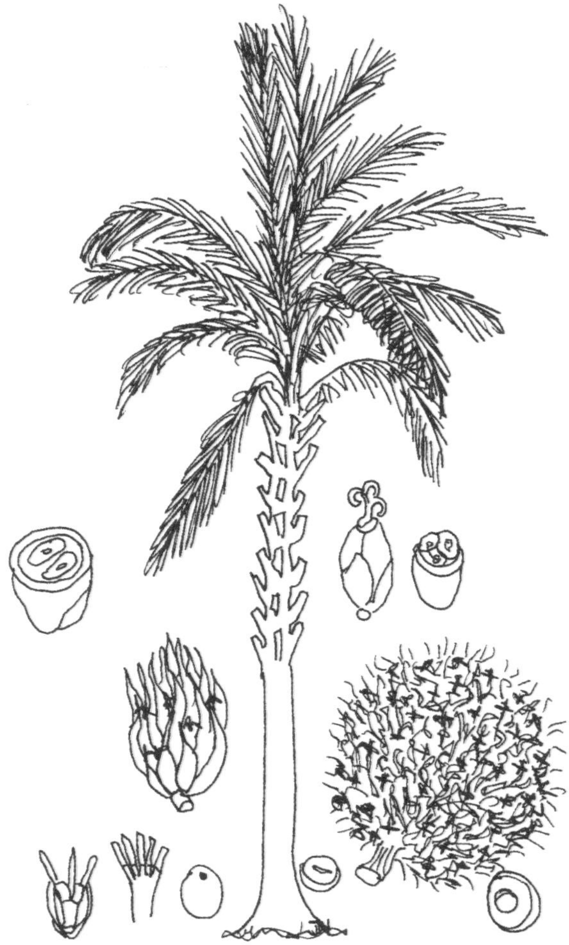

Palm oil tree

Palm oil

Like many people, I consciously avoid buying products that contain palm oil, but I am also aware that palm is only part of our problem – which is that we consume far too much fat and oil in general.

In recent years, we've learned a lot more about the health effects of various fats. The unhealthiest of these is trans-fat, which is artificially created by passing hydrogen through oils to cause them to emulsify. Partially hydrogenated oil, used in many processed baked goods and snacks and for frying foods, is a major source of trans-fat.

Many food manufacturers and restaurants have stopped using trans-fats and are looking for alternatives. One of them is palm oil; it's less saturated than butter and contains no trans-fat. But just because it's not as bad as trans-fat doesn't make it a health food.

Palm oil is made from the fruit of the oil palm tree and is one of the most widely produced edible fats in the world. Palm oil is a super-efficient crop, meaning a lot more palm oil can be grown per area of land compared to other oil crops like soybean oil or coconut oil. However, palm oil production is said to have been responsible for about 8 per cent of the world's deforestation between 1990 and 2008. And there is an associated loss of species such as orangutans, so people who are interested in issues around the environment and species diversity need to find alternatives to palm oil. However, an alternative such as coconut oil comes with its own problems, as mangrove forests are cleared in the process of growing these trees.

Palm oil is semi-solid at room temperature but can be processed into a liquid cooking oil. In general, the higher the saturated fat content, the more solid a fat is at room temperature. Coconut oil has 85 per cent saturated fat while palm oil has 50 per cent, and saturated fats are thought to be a contributory factor in blocked arteries and heart disease. For a healthier choice you could look at sunflower, rapeseed or olive oil.

Certain supermarkets say they are phasing out the use of palm oil, but then we are left with the thorny problem of what can we eat that does not entail suffering somewhere – whether it is soya in South America or huge-scale growing of sunflowers throughout France.

Meat

It has been predicted that as the world population reaches nine billion people by 2050 a dietary protein will have to be acquired by other means than animals.

As a nation we eat too much meat for our digestive systems to deal with – and too much for the Earth. One response has been a recent move to industrially producing meat-like proteins made from cloned animal cells.

For many of us, meat is nutritious, tasty and satisfying, and it is also easy to cook. The best that ethical meat eaters can do is to spend about the same amount of money but eat much less meat while choosing to source the meat from local organic or free-range farmers who love their animals and their jobs. Buying straight from the farmer would also be good for all concerned.

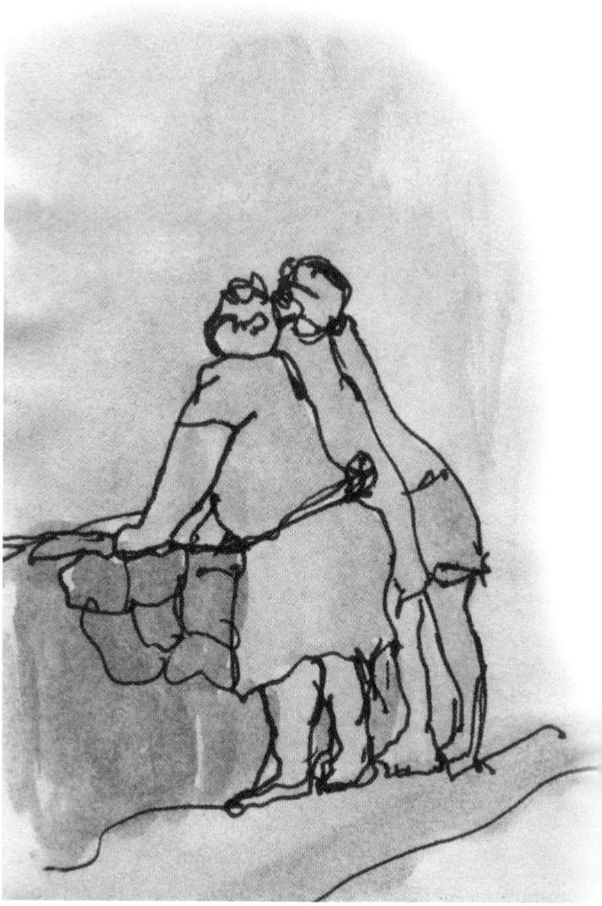

Maddy

Maddy runs an upland sheep farm with over 200 wild Welsh sheep. She knows them all and has names for many, even though they are free to roam for miles. The meat is lean and tender and tastes of the mountain herbs they have been eating. There are many people with small farms who are not contracted to large companies and supermarkets, so they have the freedom to produce happy animals but not much income. To support them would also be supporting local poor economies and traditional farming practices.

Fish

Once upon a time there were so many fish that fish was a food of the poor. Beef and oysters were served together in pies or stews, where the oysters were the bulking agent. Cod was also so plentiful that it was said you could walk across a river mouth on their backs and not get wet feet. Cod became a staple of slave plantations and in the West Indies they still refer to salted cod as provisions. Now fish stocks have been depleted worldwide through over-fishing. Factory ships hoover up fish and dredge the ocean bed, which damages deep-water habitats. Fish are no longer an endless resource.

An old friend, Lyndon won't eat fish because he does not want to contribute to the plundering of the oceans. Fish farms are not the answer to this problem, as the concentration of fish stocks leads to overcrowding and diseases, which leak out of the farm to the surrounding seas infecting the wild population. And there is also effluent pollution from some fish farms. But I need fish in my diet, especially oily fish, and especially in late summer – it is as though my brain is being switched on by whatever micro-ingredients, proteins and fats I get from mackerel or sea trout. To get a balance, I eat fish sparingly and tastily. Tinned pilchards and mackerel are so fresh when they are prepared and packed that they retain much of their goodness. Their flavour is strong enough to need just a little to stand up in curry or pie, which can be bulked out with lentils or vegetables. I buy local rod-caught fish when I can.

Raj

Raj was raised as a vegetarian, although the family ate fish occasionally. When he was 15, he would eat meat with his friends outside the home, almost as an act of rebellion. But he also admits he was interested in meat aesthetically. After reading The Hobbit, he would hold up his corn on the cob and pretend he was a troll eating a leg of mutton!

'Mutton yesterday, mutton today, and blimey, if it don't look like mutton again tomorrer,' said one of the trolls.

The Hobbit, J. R. R. Tolkien

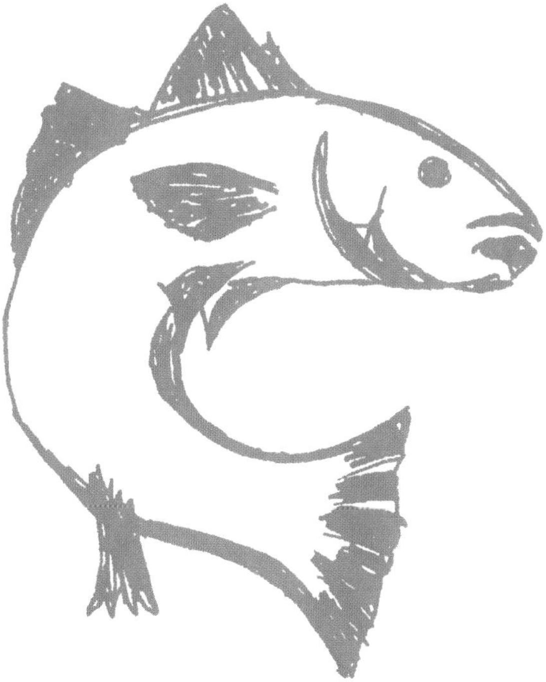

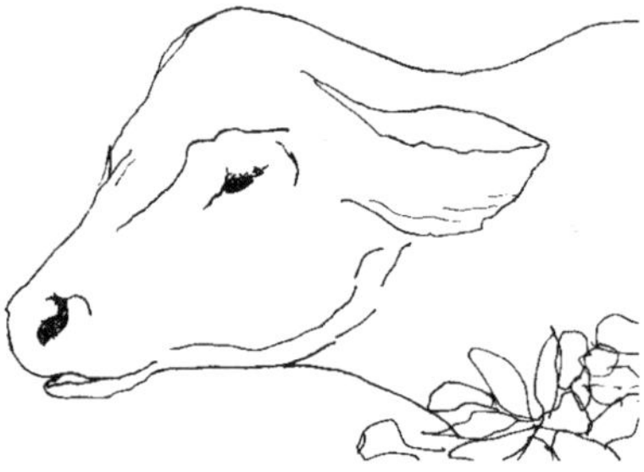

Let's have fewer calves and less milk, let's have less meat.

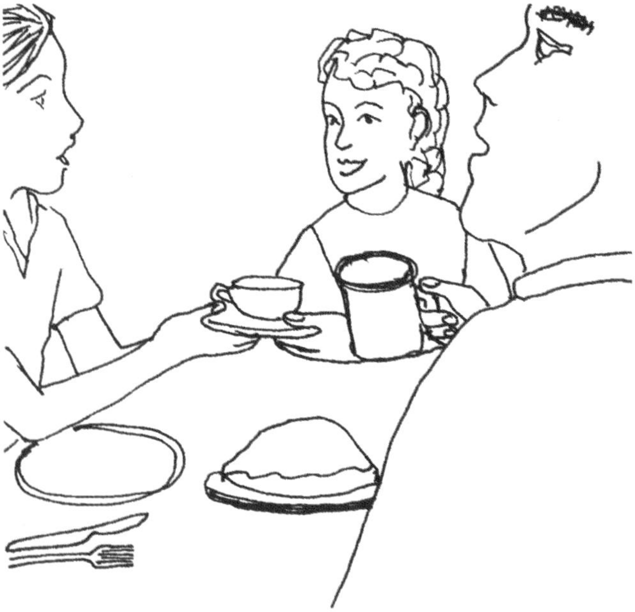

Would you like tea?

Would you like to support the dairy industry?

Dairy

According to the World Wide Fund for Nature (WWF), there are approximately 278 million dairy cows globally and the average dairy cow uses almost 500 gallons of water each day taking into account drinking water, the amount used growing feed, washing down dairy units and sterilizing equipment. Milk production also produces substantial amounts of greenhouse gas – from emissions by the cows themselves and their manure – which has a considerable effect on climate change.

Since the production and distribution of meat and milk products affect the environment through deforestation, noxious emissions and intensive use of resources like petroleum, some people avoid dairy products as a way of making an individual contribution to preserving the environment and the quality of the Earth's soil, water and air.

As well as this, many people do not want to support the treatment that the animals receive in factory farms. They don't want to drink milk and eat other dairy products that come from these sources because, by doing so, they indirectly support the farmed meat industry.

If you are concerned about the impact of dairy and meat farming on the environment but don't wish to give up dairy entirely, buy less, buy organic and buy local.

Do I get the organic, that has travelled thousands of miles, or local produce loaded with pesticides? Maybe I should join my local orchard group instead.

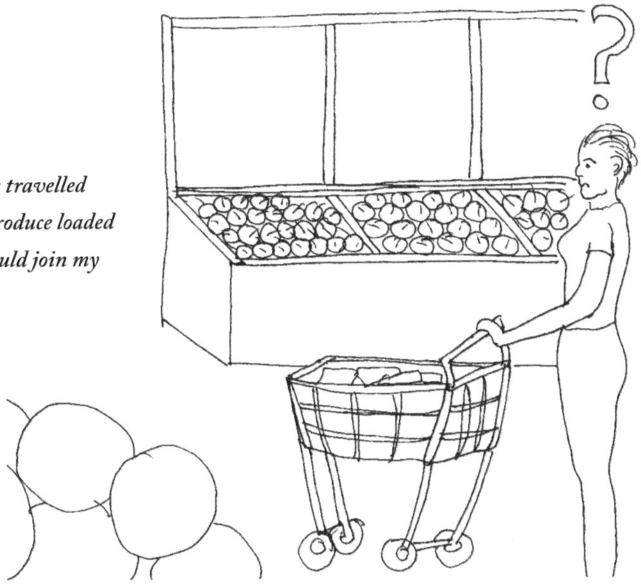

Pesticides

In 2019 six new pesticides were given licences for commercial use in polytunnels that grow soft fruit.

When I was a schoolgirl, I read Rachel Carson's book Silent Spring, which is about pesticides, their persistence in nature after their first intended use and the consequences of this. The book's title came about because of the lack of birdsong that drew Rachel Carson's attention to one effect of DDT (dichloro-diphenyl-trichloroethane – a synthetic insecticide), that led to the death of many songbirds. This chemical softened eggshells so the birds' chicks did not hatch. After I left home for university, the facts I read in this book led me to look for organic foods, which were hard to find in those days before labelling was required. When I was older and started a garden, I chose to grow organically and joined the Henry Doubleday Research Association or HDRA (now called Garden Organic), a charity that encourages people to grow organically for a healthy and sustainable world.

It stands to reason that anything that is poisonous enough to kill unwanted pests could be harmful to me, and if it is persistent then it will remain in the soil and become concentrated over the seasons.

The science behind all of this is online and is disputed or sometimes even ignored – as is anything that questions the motives or behaviour of big businesses, especially the oil and agrochemical industries. However, we are coming to realise that many species are disappearing – from insects (bees and butterflies) to mammals.

So why talk of this in a cookery book? Well, it is said that one of the reasons we have so many more sensitivities to foodstuffs now is because our bodies are actually rejecting these chemicals.

Some vegetables are said to be made acceptable by topping and tailing and peeling – potatoes, carrots, onions, for instance. Others that soak up sprays like sponges can be avoided, like broccoli, cauliflowers and lettuces. But sometimes it is better to eat these foods only a little and infrequently, buy organic or grow your own. Even on an inside windowsill you can grow your own basil, parsley and coriander, rather than buy pots that may have pesticides.

Homegrown organic apples, pears and plums are far superior to the ones that have been kept artificially almost ripe for nine months or up to a year, through a mix of pesticides, hormone retardants and protective atmospheres.

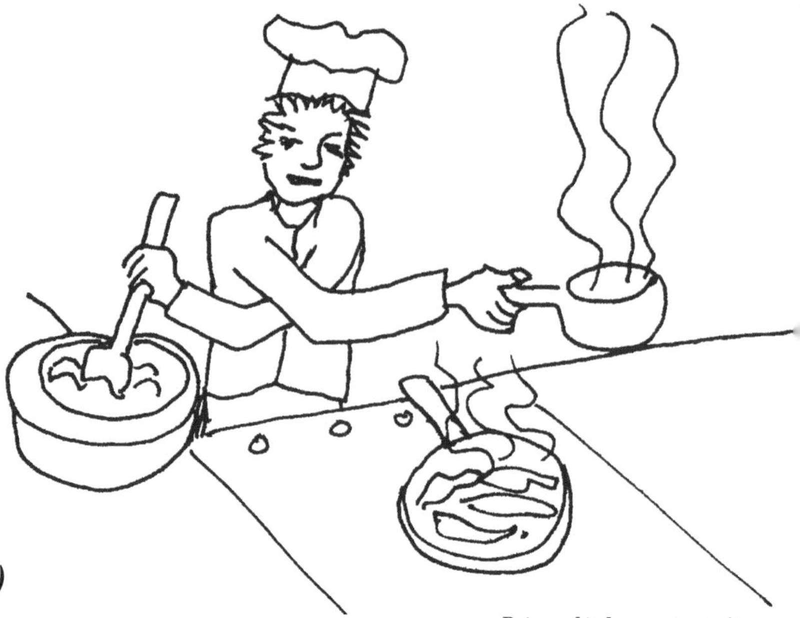

Being a kitchen genius isn't all it's cracked up to be!

Anglesey eggs (Wyau Sir Fon)

moderate oven & grill

serves 4

Serve this as an alternative to fish pie. For an inclusive feast you could also make Anglesey No Eggs (see page 22) for those who don't eat eggs.

- *450g (1lb) leeks*
- *6 hard-boiled eggs, peeled*
- *475ml (16fl oz) white or cheese sauce (see right)*
- *1 tbsp finely chopped rosemary or parsley*
- *1kg (2¼lb) potatoes or cauliflower, boiled and mashed*
- *50g (2oz) Cheddar or manchego cheese, grated (optional)*
- *salt and pepper*

Chop the leeks into 5cm (2in) rings, pop into a pan, put the lid on and steam them for about 10 minutes or until softened. Season and transfer them in the bottom of a deep baking dish.

Heat the oven to 180°C/ fan160°C/350°F/Gas 4. Halve the eggs lengthways, place them on top and cover all with sauce. Top with the mashed potatoes or cauliflower and bake for 30 minutes or until warmed through.

Remove from the oven, and then, if you like, cover with the grated cheese and grill for 5–10 minutes or until the top is golden brown.

Cheesy white sauce

stove top

serves 4

This can be used in Anglesey Eggs (see left) or as a topping for steamed vegetables. If you prefer it without the cheese, you can just omit it.

- *25g (1oz) oil, butter or your preferred substitute*
- *25g (1oz) plain or buckwheat flour*
- *300ml (½ pint) milk or your preferred substitute*
- *75–100g (3–3½oz) strong Cheddar or manchego cheese, grated*
- *salt and pepper*

Heat the oil or butter in a pan, then remove from heat and stir in the flour. Return to the heat for 3–4 minutes, stirring until it binds (to make a roux). Do not let it brown.

Remove from the heat and beat the milk in a little at a time until smooth. Return to the heat and bring to the boil, then simmer for 2 minutes, stirring all the while.

Remove from the heat, add the cheese and beat until smooth and melted.

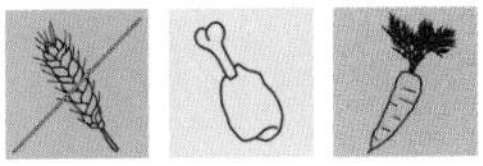

Gluten-free gravy

stove top

serves 4

This versatile gravy recipe can be used in many of the dishes in this section.

- *oil in roasting tin from your roast*
- *500ml (18fl oz) water or stock*
- *1 tbsp gluten-free flour or cornflour*
- *1 tsp tamari sauce (optional)*
- *salt and pepper*

On the hob, warm the oil in the baking tin and add the liquid, scraping the roasted remains into it to add flavour.

In a small bowl, mix the flour or cornflour with a little cold water and whisk it into the gravy as you add it. Bring to the boil, simmer and adjust the seasoning. If you prefer a thicker gravy, use more flour.

Serve in a warmed jug.

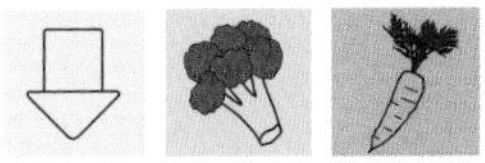

Oat & rosemary stuffing

serves 4

Make enough for vegans and vegetarians as well as meat-eaters – prepare their recipes beforehand to preclude contamination. You can use this stuffing for vegetables such as pumpkin, marrow and peppers or for meat such as turkey or rolled lamb.

- *300g (10oz) porridge oats*
- *1 medium onion, finely chopped*
- *4 tbsp sunflower or similar oil + 1 tsp for oiling tray*
- *3 tbsp finely chopped rosemary*
- *salt and pepper*

Mix everything together in a bowl using your hands. Add more oil or oats as necessary.

Bake this in an oiled tray for 20 minutes or add extra 20 minutes cooking time, if you are stuffing a roast.

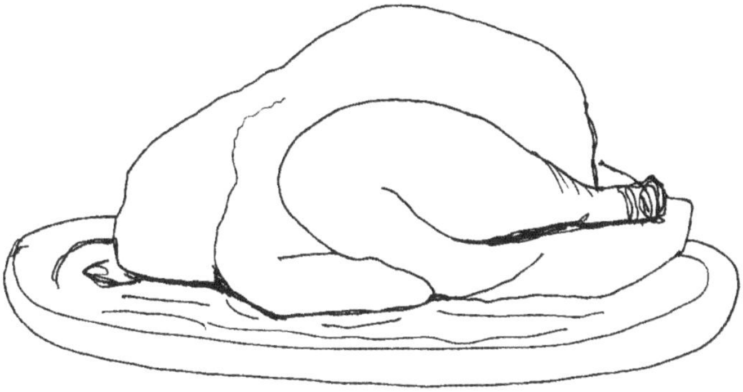

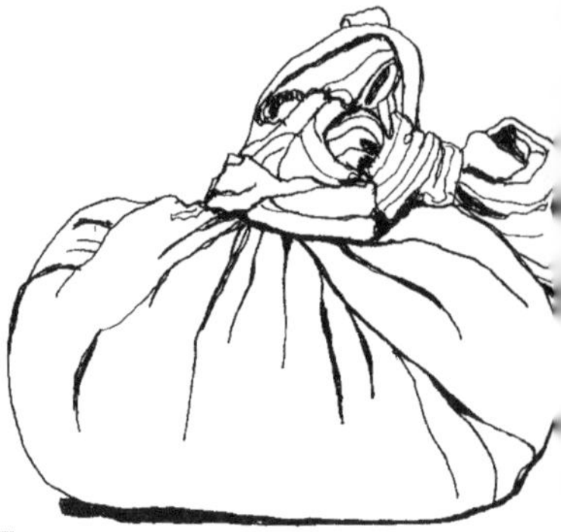

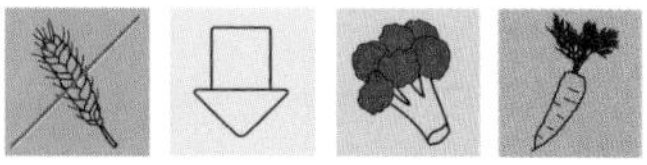

Oven-dried tomatoes

slow oven

A great lift to any vegan or vegetarian dish providing lovely umami flavour.

- *20 small ripe homegrown or organic tomatoes*
- *1 tbsp olive oil*
- *1 tsp dried basil*
- *salt and pepper*

Heat the oven to 140°C/ fan120°C/275°F/Gas 1.

Halve the tomatoes and place them face down in an oiled ceramic oven dish. Scatter over the herbs and season. Bake in the oven for 3–4 hours or until they become wrinkly and soft.

Eat or freeze in small batches to add to soups, stews and sauces as needed.

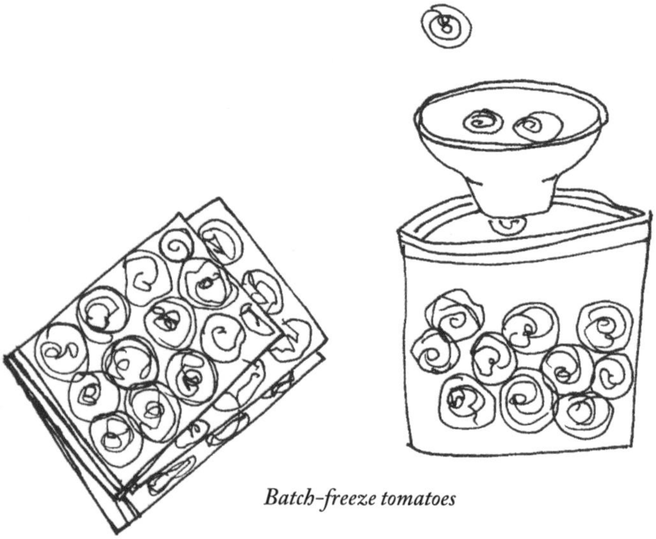

Batch-freeze tomatoes

Veggis (vegan haggis)

stove top

serves 4

There are a few commercial vegan haggis available, but they often contain palm oil. Choose this recipe to celebrate Burn's Night along with meat-eating friends. Serve with boiled neeps and tatties (turnips and potatoes).

- *1 onion, finely chopped*
- *225g (8oz) Sosmix (vegetarian sausage mix) or chestnut stuffing (see page 91)*
- *1 tbsp chopped rosemary*
- *1 tbsp chopped sage*
- *1 tsp ground white pepper*
- *125g (4oz) oatmeal (steel cut oats)*
- *125g (4oz) rolled oats*
- *1 tbsp oil + 1 tbsp for greasing pudding basin*
- *500ml (18fl oz) stock or water*
- *salt and pepper*

In a bowl, mix together all the ingredients and stir well. Stuff the mix into a greased pudding basin. Cover the top with a large square of greaseproof paper and tin foil.

If using a pudding cloth, place the pudding mix on a square of greaseproof paper in the centre of the cloth and bring the edges of paper and the cloth together before wrapping and tying it tightly.

Whichever method you use, place the pudding on a steamer rack in a pan with a tightly fitting lid and steam for 2 hours until firm and well cooked.

Haggis

stove top

serves 4

There are some good organic commercial haggis available though they may contain more offal than you would want, such as lambs offal (heart, liver, kidneys) with unnamed beef offal. Choose Veggis for a vegan recipe.

- *2 onions, finely chopped*
- *1 lamb's liver, finely chopped*
- *1 lamb's heart, finely chopped*
- *350g (12oz) minced lamb*
- *1 tbsp dried mixed herbs*
- *125g (4½oz) oatmeal (steel cut oats)*
- *125g (4½oz) rolled oats*
- *125g (4½oz) suet*
- *110ml (4fl oz) stock or water*
- *1 washed sheep's stomach or follow Veggis recipe (see page 116) to use a pudding cloth*
- *salt and pepper, to taste*

Mix together all the ingredients (apart from the stomach) and add enough of the stock or water to soften the mix. Stuff the mix into the washed sheep's stomach, and seal with some kitchen string to prevent the filling escaping. Wrap in foil and place in a pan of simmering water. Simmer for 1–2 hours until firm and well cooked. Test it with meat thermometer, as for roast lamb.

Serve hot with boiled neeps and tatties (turnips and potatoes).

Raw stuffed courgette (zucchini) flowers

per person

A simple dish to bring a sense of luxury to your table in mixed company. Serve as hors d'oeuvre or side dish with raw food dishes.

- *2 tbsp nut, tofu or sunflower seed cream (do not use vanilla or sugar to make the cream)*
- *1 tsp each of lemon zest and juice*
- *1 tsp finely chopped thyme, basil, rosemary, marjoram or mint*
- *2 courgette (zucchini) flowers*
- *salt and pepper*

Combine the nut, tofu or sunflower seed cream with the lemon and herbs and seasoning. Stuff the flowers with the mixture and serve immediately.

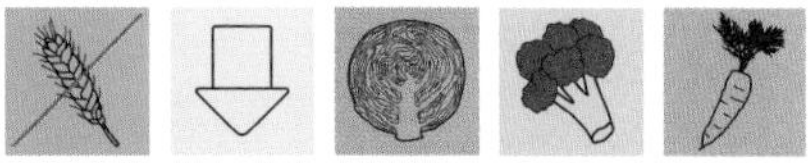

Cauliflower rice

per person

This is a quickly made dish which looks delightful for people who follow a raw diet. As an alternative, try using spiralised courgette (zucchini) and finely chopped cauliflower.

- *75g (3oz) finely grated cauliflower*
- *25g (1oz) finely chopped courgette (zucchini)*
- *25g (1oz) finely chopped carrot*
- *25g (1oz) finely chopped onion (optional)*
- *25g (1oz) finely chopped cucumber*
- *1 tsp finely chopped basil*
- *2 tsp fresh lemon or lime juice*
- *salt and pepper*

Make a ring with the grated cauliflower on a plate. Mix the rest of the ingredients together and pile inside the ring finishing with the basil leaves and citrus juice. Season to taste and serve immediately.

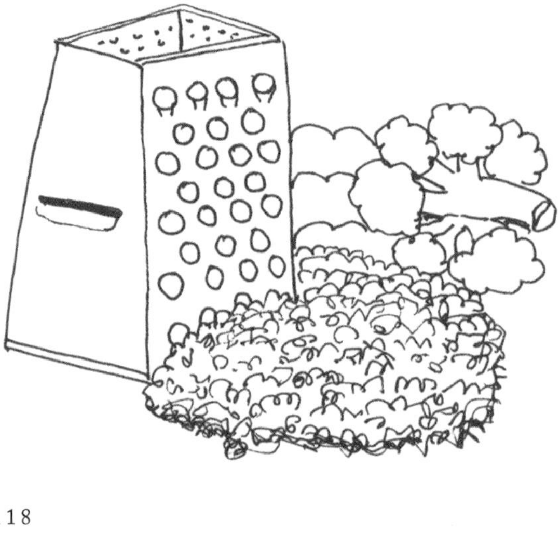

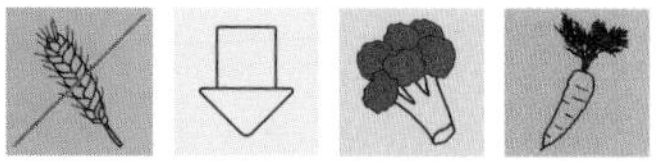

Perfect roast potatoes

hot oven

per person

Many of the dishes in this section go with potatoes and this is one of those perfect recipes. Some people peel potatoes, some scrub. Either way this makes scrumptious roasties.

- *2–3 potatoes per person, cut into 3–4cm (1¼–1½in) cubes*
- *2 tbsp gluten-free or buckwheat flour*
- *5 tbsp hot oil*
- *salt and pepper*

Heat the oven to 180°C/ fan160°C/350°F/Gas 4.

Put the potatoes into a pan of boiling water and parboil for about 10 minutes, or until just done. Drain, shaking the potatoes in the colander to roughen up the edges, then return to the pan and leave to cool for 5 minutes. Put a roasting pan with the oil in the oven to heat through.

Drench the potatoes with the flour and season. Tip the potatoes into the roasting tin, shake it vigorously until all are well covered in the hot oil, then roast in the oven for 30–40 minutes or until golden brown and crispy.

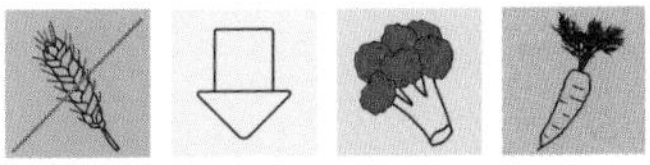

Tempura vegetables

stove top

serves 4

Tempura is quick to make and versatile enough to be a main or a side dish for a feast. Make these first if you are using the same oil to make the seafood version.

Tempura Batter

- *85g (3oz) plain gluten-free flour*
- *½ tsp salt*
- *½ tsp sugar*
- *200ml (7fl oz) sparkling water*

Vegetables

- *50g (2oz) plain gluten-free flour*
- *225g (8oz) mix of finely sliced vegetables – courgette (zucchini), red pepper, mushrooms, carrots*
- *oil, for deep-frying*

In a bowl, whisk all the batter ingredients together to a watery thin liquid.

Heat the oil in a wok or deep pan.

Add the flour to a bowl and dip the vegetables one at a time into it until coated on all sides, tapping off any excess, then dip them into the tempura batter. Shake off any drips.

Test the temperature of the oil by dropping a piece of battered vegetable into the pan – if it sizzles it is ready. Batch-fry the vegetables until the batter is golden brown and crispy.

Serve hot with dipping sauces and chopped coriander.

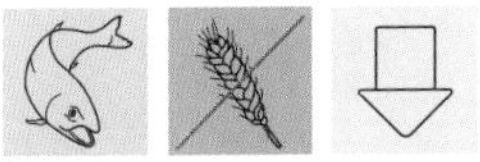

Tempura seafood

stove top

serves 4

After many years without one, my hometown now has a fish shop which stocks sustainably sourced and locally caught fish. Their sea mix makes a perfect blend for tempura. Shop locally if you are able.

Tempura Batter

- *85g (3oz) plain gluten-free flour*
- *½ tsp salt*
- *½ tsp sugar*
- *200ml (7fl oz) sparkling water, chilled*

Seafood

- *50g (2oz) plain gluten-free flour*
- *225g (8oz) mix of seafood and filleted fish strips*
- *oil, for deep-frying*

In a bowl, whisk all the batter ingredients together to a watery thin liquid.

Heat the oil in a wok or deep pan.

Add the flour to a bowl and dip the seafood pieces and fish into it until coated on all sides, tapping off any excess, then dip them into the tempura batter. Shake off any drips.

Test the temperature of the oil by dropping a piece of battered seafood into the pan – if it sizzles it is ready. Batch-fry the seafood until the batter is golden brown and crispy.

Drain and serve hot with dipping sauces and chopped corriander (cilantro).

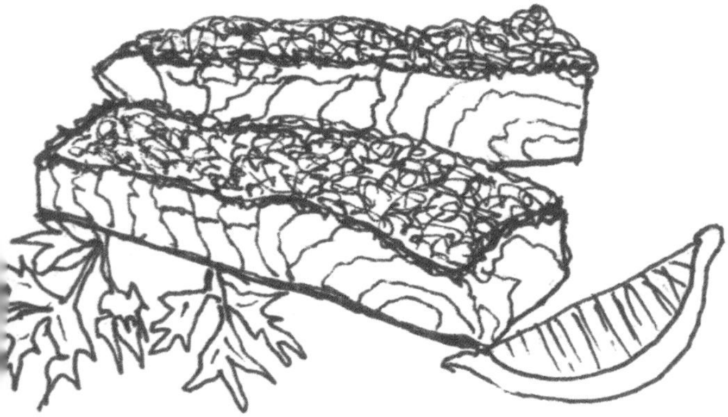

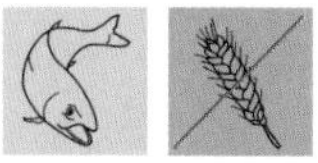

Fish with herby crust

moderate oven

per person

If you are planning a meaty feast day, this is a good alternative fish dish.

- *1 tbsp olive oil*
- *1 tbsp fresh gluten-free or spelt breadcrumbs*
- *1 tbsp chopped herbs – mix of thyme, rosemary, marjoram*
- *180g (6oz) skinless and boneless white fish steak*
- *salt and pepper*

Heat the oven to 180°C/ fan160°C/350°F/Gas 4.

Add the oil to the herbs and breadcrumbs, season and mix well.

Place the fish on a baking tray and spread the mix evenly on top. Bake for 10–15 minutes until the top is golden and the fish is flaky and cooked through.

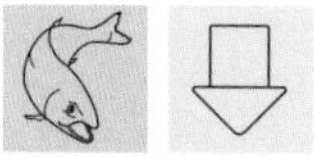

Fish pie

stove top & moderate oven

serves 4

A staple of British cuisine and loved by all pescatarians.

- *450g (1lb) mix of fish pieces (whitefish, salmon, prawns, smoked haddock)*
- *350ml (12fl oz) milk or your preferred substitute*
- *40g (1½oz) flour or cornflour*
- *1 tbsp finely chopped parsley*
- *100ml (3½fl oz) cream or soya cream*
- *6 hard-boiled eggs, peeled and halved*
- *450g (1lb) warm mashed potatoes or cauliflower*
- *salt and pepper*

Heat the oven to 180°C/ fan160°C/350°F/Gas 4.

Put the fish pieces in a pan with the liquid and simmer for about 3 minutes or until just cooked through.

Drain off the liquid and use this to make a simple white sauce. In a cup, mix a little of the liquid with the flour or cornflour. Heat the rest of the milk in a pan until almost boiling. Remove from the heat and whisk in the flour mix, then return to the heat and stir continuously until boiling. Season to taste and stir in the parsley and cream.

Place the fish in a baking dish. Arrange the egg halves on top. Cover with the sauce and top with the mash.

Cook in the oven for about 15 minutes or until thoroughly warmed through. Then if you like grill the top until brown and crusty. Serve with peas and salad.

Lamb casserole

oven

serves 4

One of the simplest and easiest ways to prepare a tasty lamb supper. Try adding 1 tablespoon of Moroccan spice and a tin of chickpeas when cooking and serve with flatbreads.

- *450g (1lb) diced lamb*
- *1 tbsp oil*
- *2 onions, chopped*
- *3 carrots, chopped*
- *2 parsnips or swedes, chopped (optional)*
- *500ml (18fl oz) stock*
- *1 tbsp tamari*
- *1 tbsp finely chopped rosemary*
- *salt and pepper*

Heat the oven to 180°C/ fan160°C/350°F/Gas 4.

Fry the lamb in the oil in a casserole dish until the outsides are golden brown, then remove the lamb and set it to one side. Fry the onions and carrots in the oil from the lamb.

Return the lamb to the casserole with the vegetables and cover with the stock. Add the tamari and rosemary and seasoning.

Cook in the oven for 2 hours. Serve with warm bread and steamed cabbage.

Mini meatloaf

hot oven

serves 4

Most commercial meat loaves contain preservatives such as sodium nitrite and sodium nitrate and there is no provenance to the meat. This recipe allows you to choose exactly what to include and is super tasty.

- *450g (1lb) minced lamb or pork*
- *1 large onion, finely chopped*
- *1 egg*
- *1 carrot, grated*
- *1 garlic clove, minced*
- *1 tbsp finely chopped sage*
- *1 tbsp tamari, kelp powder or bouillon to taste*
- *4 tbsp gluten-free, buckwheat or wholemeal flour*
- *salt and pepper*

Heat the oven to 200°C/ fan180°C/400°F/Gas 6.

Using your hands, combine all the ingredients except the flour in a large mixing bowl.

Put the flour on a plate and use it and your floury hands to form the mix into little loaves and place them on a baking tray, or press into silicon muffin trays.

Bake for 30 minutes, then serve hot or cold.

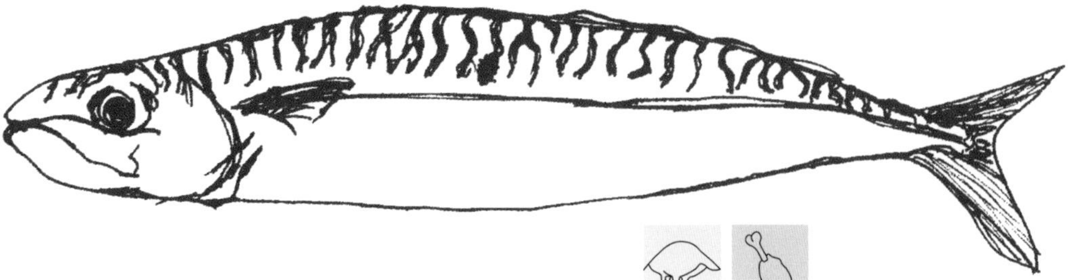

BBQ mackerel

barbeque

per person

Barbecues are often synonymous with burgers and chops, so it's good to offer a simple and delicious fish alternative.

- *1 gutted mackerel*
- *lemon wedges, to serve*
- *salt and pepper*

Lay the mackerel on a hot barbecue or griddle pan and cook for 5–8 minutes one each side or until the skin is charred and the flesh is firm but cooked through.

Remove from the heat and season lightly.

Serve with gremolata (page 95) and a lemon wedge.

Tip: Alternatively, mackerel is easy to cook in the oven. Place the seasoned fish in a baking tray with a little oil. Cover and bake in the oven at 200°C/ fan180°C/400°F/Gas 6 for 15–20 minutes. Serve as above.

Strong pastry

serves 4

Pasties are traditionally made using strong pastry. So if you are happy to eat lard and dairy, here is the recipe I use. For an alternative choose GF pastry (see page 78). Make this in advance of your recipe so it can rest for 3 hours before using.

- *450g (1lb) strong white flour*
- *1 tsp salt*
- *120g (4oz) lard, cut into cubes*
- *125g (4½oz) butter, cut into cubes*
- *150ml (5fl oz) cold water*

Sift together the flour and salt into a large mixing bowl. Rub the cubes of lard and butter into the flour with your fingertips until it resembles breadcrumbs. Little by little pour in the cold water, mixing it in, until it forms a binding dough. Knead until the pastry in the bowl becomes elastic.

Wrap the ball of pastry in cling film and leave in the fridge to rest for 3 hours.

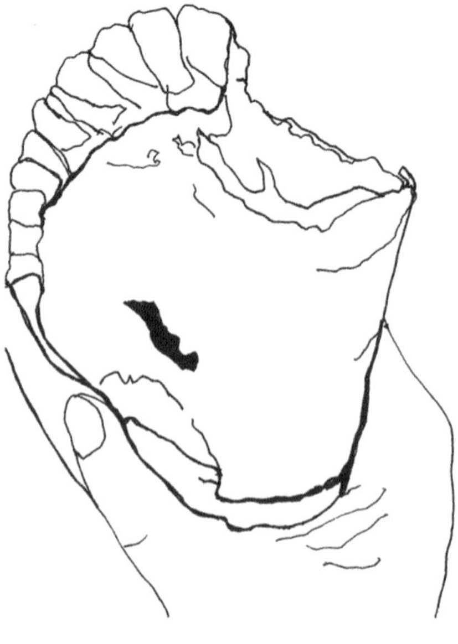

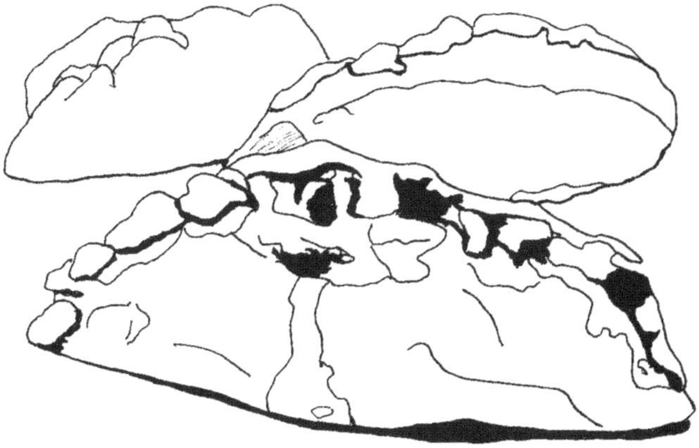

Curried vegetable pasties

oven

serves 4

These make a good alternative to traditional Cornish pasties and can be made using leftover curried vegetables.

- *450g (1lb) butternut squash, peeled and cut into 1–2cm (¼in to ½in) cubes*
- *2 medium carrots, chopped*
- *2 medium onions, finely sliced*
- *2 tbsp oil*
- *2 garlic cloves, pressed*
- *300ml (10fl oz) water*
- *2 tbsp of mild curry powder or 2 tsp ground coriander, ground cumin or turmeric, or*
- *cardamom pods, ¼ tsp chilli flakes, or to taste*
- *1 tbsp finely chopped coriander (cilantro)*
- *350g (12oz) Strong pastry (see left) made with vegan margarine*
- *flour, for dusting*
- *milk or milk substitute to glaze*
- *salt and pepper*

Mix all the filling ingredients together except for the spices and coriander, and simmer for 10–20 minutes in a pan filled with the water until the vegetables are just soft – add more water if needed and cook longer for a mushy mix.

Adjust the seasoning, adding the curry powder and coriander, and cool for 10 minutes.

Heat the oven to 180°C/ fan160°C/350°F/Gas 4.

Roll out the pastry on a floured work surface to a depth of ½cm (¼in) and cut into 20cm (8in) discs. Make a small pile in the middle of each circle of pastry. Bring the top over, fold down the edges and crimp tightly, in a Cornish pasty shape. Glaze with milk substitute or beaten egg.

Bake for 30 minutes in the oven until golden brown and cooked through.

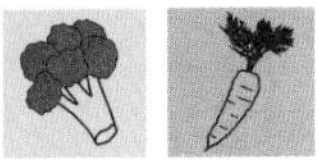

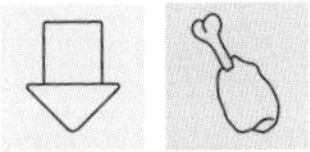

Cornish pasties

oven

serves 4

Historic British pasties are popularly sold online from companies in Cornwall. There is a growing list of variations such as cheese and mushroom or chicken. Here you can cook the traditional mix or decide exactly what you would like in your pasty.

- *350g (12oz) Strong pastry (see left)*
- *flour, for dusting*
- *450g (1lb) cubed beef skirt*
- *350g (12oz) potatoes, peeled and diced*
- *150g (5oz) swede or turnip, peeled and diced*
- *150g (5oz) onion, peeled and sliced*
- *milk or milk substitute or beaten egg, to glaze*
- *salt and pepper*

Heat the oven to 180°C/ fan160°C/350°F/Gas 4.

Roll out the pastry on a floured work surface to a depth of ½cm (¼in) and cut into a 20cm (8in) circle for each pasty. Mix all the filling ingredients together in a large mixing bowl and pile it in the middle of the pastry circle. Bring the top over, fold down the edges and crimp tightly. Glaze with milk, milk substitute or beaten egg.

Bake in the oven for 55 minutes until golden brown and cooked through.

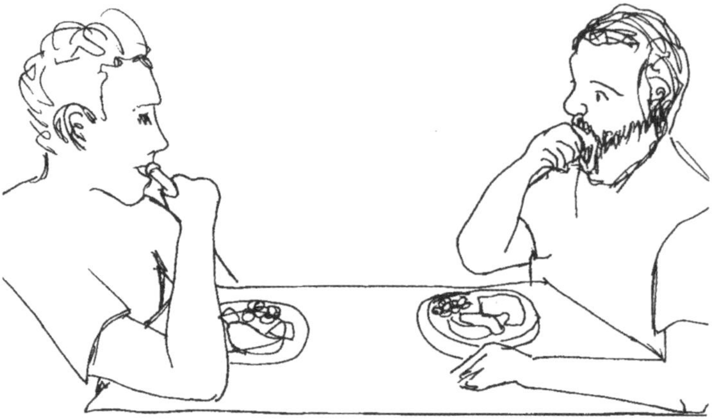

VEGETARIANS

Strict vegetarians do not eat meat, fish, poultry, gelatine jelly, animal fats (as in some margarines) or cheese containing rennet.

Vegetarians do not eat chicken, even though my mum, like many older people, thought chicken was not proper meat! They don't eat sausages or enjoy a little of the gravy off the joint.

To be vegetarian is to eat no meat products but still eat some animal foods such as dairy and eggs, while some eat fish and shellfish too.. Some people become vegetarian because they just don't like the texture or the taste of meat, some because they do not want to support the meat industry or are distressed about rain forests being destroyed to grow animal feed. Try not to point out to them that the dairy industry carries the same global guilt as the meat industry – they are your friends and family, remember.

Vegetarians, like most people, prefer strong, rich flavours, so they would be happy with a serving of Italian or Indian food. I have known some vegetarians who did not like vegetables. Many eat eggs and cheese, but it is hard on them when the alternative they are so often offered is cheese omelette.

Eating more fruit and vegetables is linked to a lower risk of getting diseases such as cancer, stroke, chronic heart disease and dying early.

Vegetables

Lots of people say we should eat more vegetables. But what are vegetables?

A vegetable is anything off a plant that is not a fruit. Though some fruits can be vegetables, it seems that no vegetables can be fruits. Unless pumpkin or carrot can be

Trish

Trish became vegetarian when she was around eight years old. Her family lived near Coventry Airport and after seeing a large protest there against the transportation of livestock she became really passionate about animal rights. She wasn't allowed to join the protest, but her mum helped her and her brother to make signs to hand out to the protesters. She has been vegetarian ever since.

Trish says, 'Given the reasons I am vegetarian, I should also be vegan. The dairy industry is as cruel as the meat industry and I am currently breastfeeding my daughter, so I feel terrible for the dairy cows. When I tried veganism for six weeks, a few years ago, I ended up eating a lot of processed food, such as vegan fish fingers and Oreos. I think to be a successful vegan, you'd need to pre-plan and do a lot of cooking. I'm just not that into cooking.'

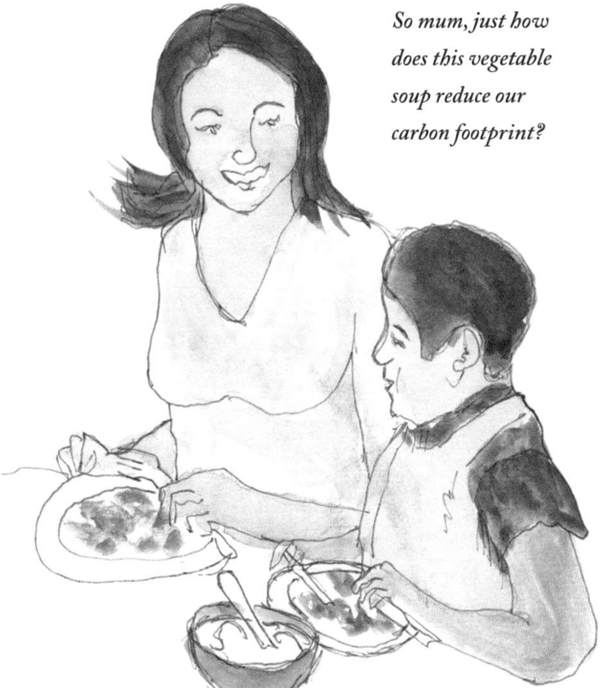

So mum, just how does this vegetable soup reduce our carbon footprint?

classed as fruits when you use them to make pumpkin pie or carrot cake… And, of course, pumpkin is a fruit which is treated as a vegetable.

Traditionally veggies are those plant foods that we eat with savoury dishes, but if you eat a tagine, you will probably have eaten apricots in it, and some pizzas have fresh figs with goat's cheese.

I keep a garden and have a rotation system that neatly divides vegetable into four kinds, so perhaps it would be best to use that to make a list:

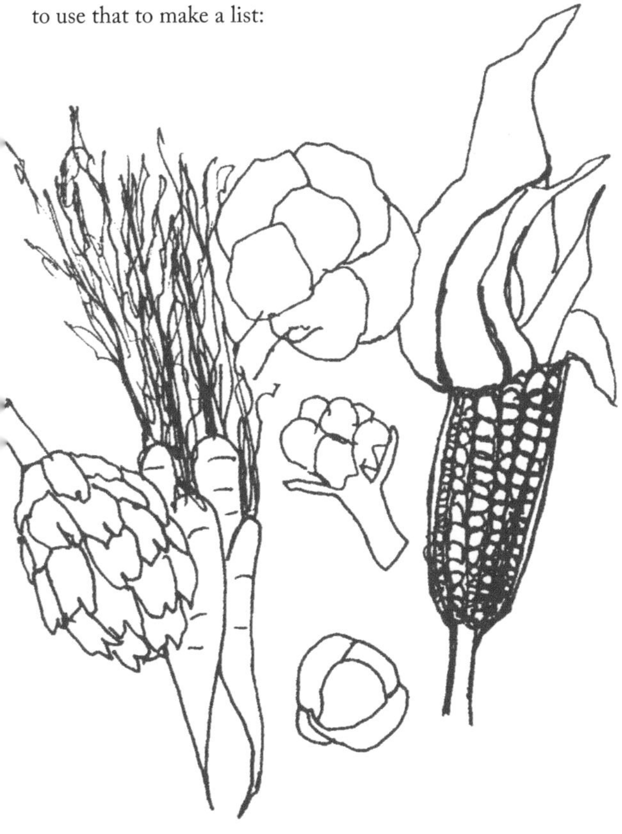

A good mix of vegetables, especially if they are home grown or locally sourced, will improve the diversity of your gut flora and can improve your overall health.

Garlic is an excellent source of vitamin B6 (pyridoxine). It is also a very good source of manganese, selenium and vitamin C.

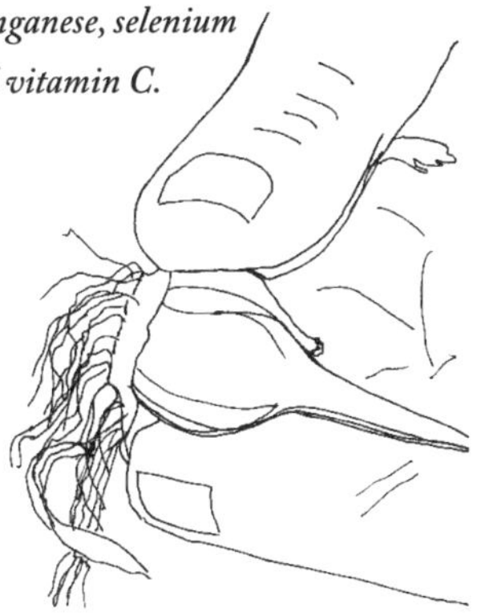

Roots

Potatoes, carrots, parsnips, swedes, turnips, Jerusalem artichokes, sweet potatoes, onions (spring, red, brown, white), shallots, garlic and leeks.

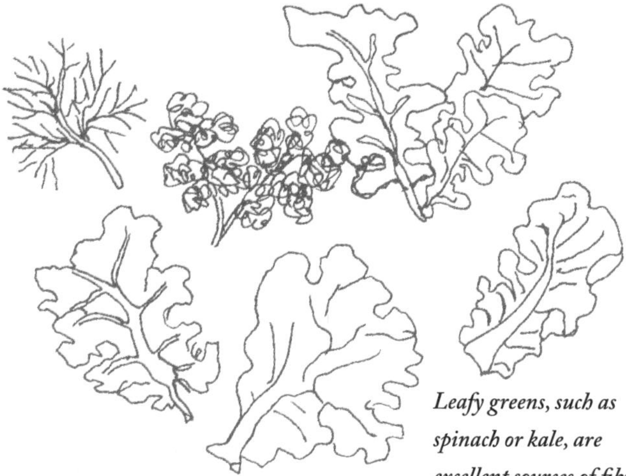

Leafy greens, such as spinach or kale, are excellent sources of fibre, as well as nutrients like folic acid (vitamin B12), vitamin C, vitamin K and vitamin A.

Leaves

All the cabbage family: sprouts, cabbages (red and white, spring), kale (red, curly, Russian, cavolo nero), cauliflower, broccoli and calabrese. The rest include spinach, chard, Florence fennel, lettuce of many sorts, rocket, chicory cress and chives.

The fibre in green beans and fresh peas, helps to keep your digestive system healthy and running smoothly.

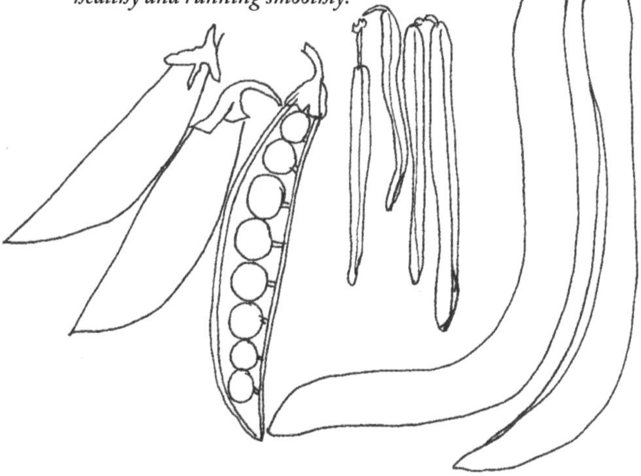

Peas & beans when fresh

Peas, mangetout, runner beans, French beans (purple and green, climbing and dwarf), broad beans and climbing flat beans.

Beans, lentils and split peas are rich in the indigestible carbohydrates that beneficial gut bacteria need.

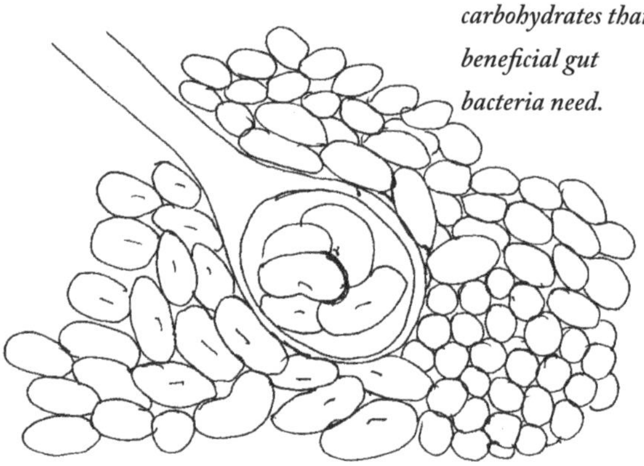

Peas & beans when dry

Marrowfat peas, lentils (red, brown, green, yellow, bijoux), black-eyed peas, black, red, haricot and kidney beans, butter beans and chickpeas.

Figs are an excellent source of prebiotics, which improve overall gut health and a good source of calcium and potassium.

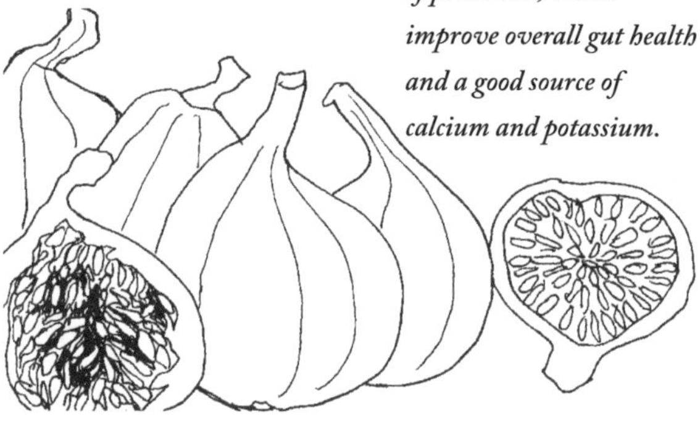

Fruits

Tomatoes (red, yellow, beef, dwarf, heritage), peppers (red, green, yellow, black, bell, pointed), aubergine, cucumber, pumpkin, squash, courgette (yellow zucchini, green) and marrow.

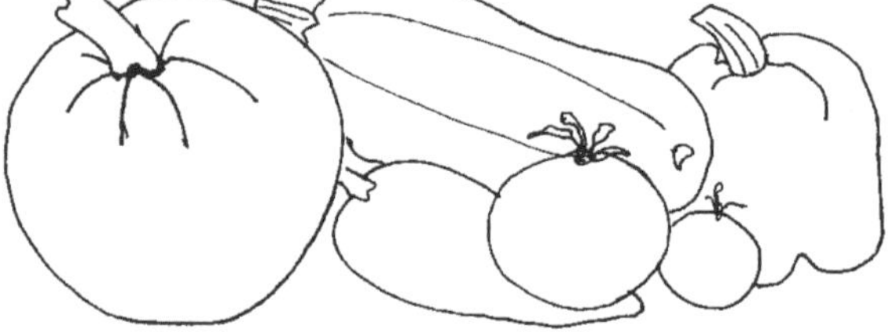

Neither plant nor animal, fungi are in a class of their own. They can boost your immune system and your brain.

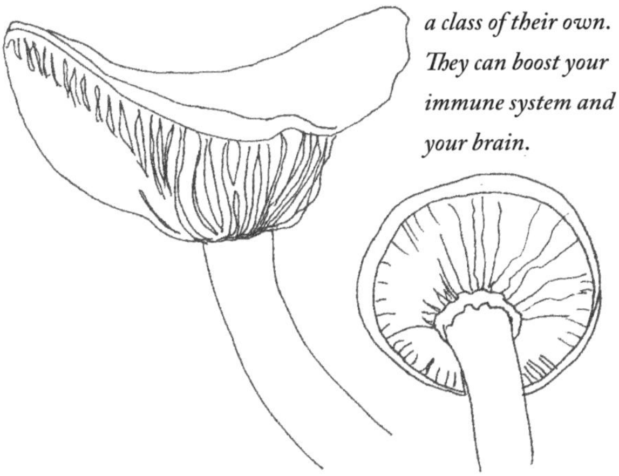

Fungi

Mushrooms (shitake, field, chestnut and button and in-season chanterelle).

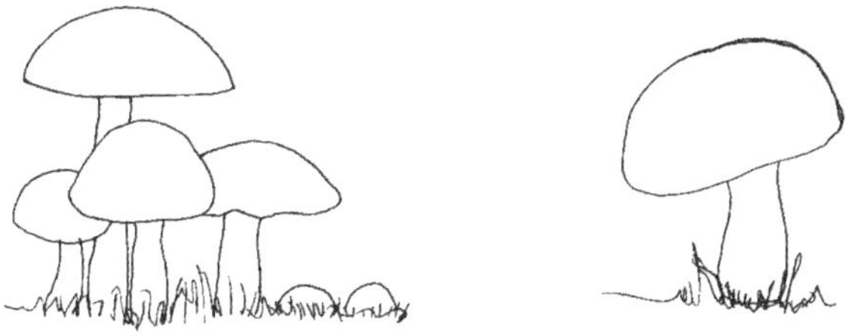

Hey, you look like a fungi, wanna come to a party?

The average meal contains only a few of all these ingredients for most of us but represents a cornucopia for vegetarians before you even begin to add fish or dairy ingredients.

The classic meat and two veg will always include potatoes as one of the veg but the other could be peas or cabbage in most households. Big breakfasts generally include tomatoes and mushrooms. Pizza, offers peppers, onions and mushrooms as toppings. Baked beans can accompany any meal and perhaps we can count tomato ketchup as one of our five a day.

Left: Colourful fruits and vegetables contribute to a healthy gut because they contain phytonutrients that promote the growth of beneficial microbial species such as Bifidobacteria and Lactobacilli.

RECIPES

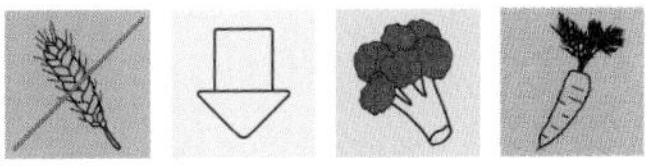

Dumplings

stove top

serves 4–6

Add these to vegetable soup (see page 138) or stew (see page 131) or even Norah's soup (see page 138) to make an evening meal.

- *225g (8oz) wholewheat or gluten-free flour, plus extra for dusting*
- *1 tsp bicarbonate of soda (baking soda) or 2 tsp baking powder*
- *1 tsp dried thyme or 2 tsp chopped fresh thyme*
- *110g (4oz) fat (cold butter or vegan spread which has been frozen so it will grate)*
- *100ml (3½fl oz) cold water*
- *salt and pepper*

Combine the first four ingredients in a bowl. Grate the cold or frozen fat into the mix. Add enough cold water, a spoonful at a time, to make a soft dough.

With well-floured hands, lightly form into golf-sized balls and place them in the liquid of the cooked stew. Cover with a lid and simmer gently for 15 minutes.

Scoop out and spoon into bowls and surround with stew.

Frittata

stove top & hot oven

per person

This is a nutritious and exotic take on an omelette.

- *1 medium potato, thinly sliced*
- *2 tbsp frying oil*
- *1 tbsp finely chopped courgette (zucchini)*
- *1 tbsp thinly sliced onion*
- *1 tbsp sliced red pepper (optional)*
- *1 mushroom, chopped*
- *2 eggs*
- *1 tsp dried mixed herbs*
- *salt and pepper*
- *25–50g (1–2oz) grated cheese for topping – vegan, feta, manchego or Cheddar*

Heat the oven to 180°C/ fan160°C/350°F/Gas 4.

Boil the potato for a few minutes until just done and drain.

In a small ovenproof frying pan, fry the vegetables in the oil until golden. Add a little more oil to the pan if needed.

Separate the eggs. Beat the yolks thoroughly and add the herbs and seasoning. Beat the whites in a bowl to form peaks. Gently fold the whites into the yolks and pour the mix onto the fried ingredients. Layer the potatoes on top and finish with cheese. Bake for 10–20 minutes until risen and golden brown.

Huevas rancheros

stove top

per person

Huevas rancheros is a traditional Mexican breakfast dish which can also be served as a colourful tasty lunch.

- *1 kale leaf, finely chopped*
- *1 tbsp finely chopped onion*
- *1 small bird's eye chilli, finely chopped (optional)*
- *1 tbsp finely chopped courgette (zucchini)*
- *1 garlic clove, finely chopped*
- *100ml (3½fl oz) tomato passata*
- *2 tsp sunflower oil*
- *2 tsp olive oil*
- *2 eggs*
- *1 tbsp chopped coriander (cilantro) leaves*
- *salt and pepper*

Mix the kale, onion, chilli, courgette and garlic together in a lidded frying pan, season and stir in the sunflower oil. Fry the mix for 5-10 minutes, with the lid on, occasionally stirring until all are softened, then add the passata and stir well.

Make a hole in the middle, pour the olive oil into the clear area and break the eggs into it. Lower the heat and, with the pan lid on, cook for 3–4 minutes until the eggs are cooked to taste.

Sprinkle with coriander leaves and serve immediately.

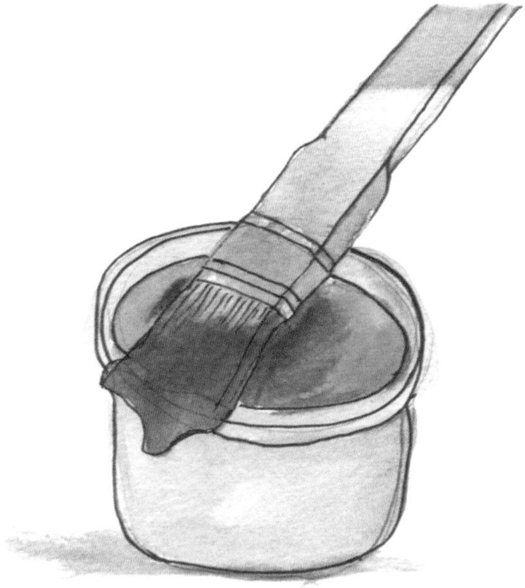

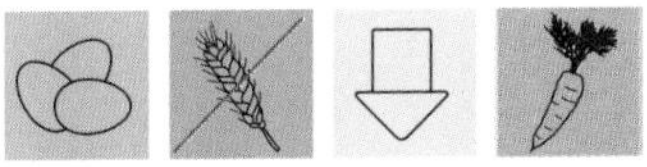

Kale & poached egg

stove top

per person

My favourite post-fasting breakfast. It has all the food values served on toasted GF, sourdough or rye bread. Try spinach as an alternative to kale.

- *1 small onion, finely chopped (optional)*
- *1 small chilli (optional)*
- *1 tbsp olive oil*
- *100g (4oz) kale (curly or dark), finely chopped*
- *1 or 2 eggs*
- *1 tsp vinegar (optional)*
- *1 toasted muffin or 2 slices toasted bread*

Sauté the onion and chilli, if using, in a pan with some olive oil. Add the kale and stir around until all is soft.

In the meantime, poach the eggs in a pan of simmering salted water. (Add 1 teaspoon of vinegar if eggs are not newly laid.)

Place the kale on the toast. Drain the eggs and place on top. Season and serve hot.

BBQ sauce

serves 4

This barbecue sauce lifts vegetarian sausages or burger to the next level. It is delicious over barbecued braised tofu as well. Use as a marinade or brush on as a basting sauce. For extra heat add 1 teaspoon of cayenne pepper or some chilli sauce.

- *4 tbsp tomato purée*
- *2 garlic cloves, finely chopped*
- *2 tbsp olive oil*
- *100ml (3½fl oz) cider vinegar*
- *1 tbsp finely grated fresh root ginger*
- *1 tbsp muscovado or coconut sugar*
- *1 tbsp tamari or soy sauce*
- *salt and pepper*

Beat together all the ingredients until smooth.

Tian of tomatoes & courgettes

oven

serves 4 as a side dish, or 1 as a main

This can be served with all the BBQ dishes or as a dish to accompany pie or pasty or baked potato and salad.

- *1 tbsp olive oil, plus 1 tsp*
- *1 courgette (zucchini), cut into 1cm (½in) slices*
- *1 beef tomato, cut into 1cm (½in) slices*
- *pinch of fresh or dried basil or thyme*
- *salt and pepper*

Heat the oven to 180°C/ fan160°C/350°F/Gas 4.

Spread the olive oil in the base of a heavy baking dish.

Lay the courgettes and tomato slices on their sides, alternating them in a spiral.

Season, top with herbs and drizzle with the teaspoon of olive oil.

Bake for 40 minutes until golden on top.

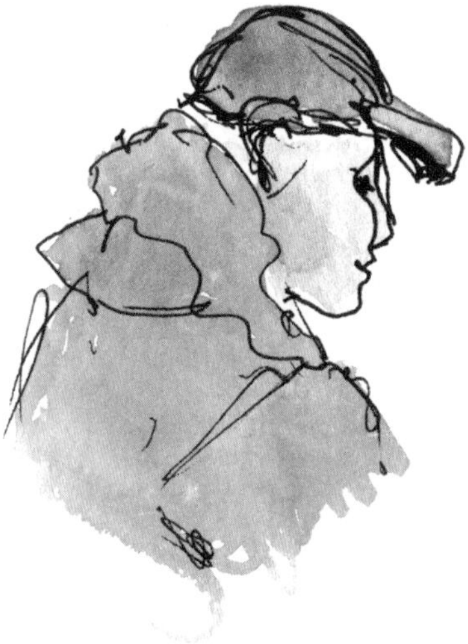

Roast vegetables

hot oven

serves 4

Perfect vegetarian fare that can be served with vegan dishes, with meat dishes or fish.

- *1kg (2¼lb) mix of red pepper, aubergine (eggplant), leek, courgette (zucchini), carrot, parsnip, onion, roughly chopped*
- *8 whole button mushrooms*
- *2 tbsp finely chopped herbs – rosemary, thyme, sage*
- *8 whole garlic cloves or 2 halved heads of garlic*
- *oil, for roasting*
- *salt and pepper*

Heat the oven to 200°C/ fan180°C/400°F/Gas 6.

Fill a roasting tin with the chopped vegetables, mushrooms, herbs and garlic. Use your hands to cover them all in oil and spread them out evenly.

Roast in a hot oven, turning occasionally until all are golden. Some veg will be crisper than others. If you would prefer them all crisp then roast the root veg for 10 minutes before adding the rest.

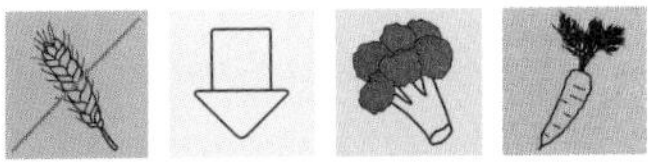

Vegetable stew

stove top

serves 4

Serve this with dumplings (see page 127) or on its own with chunks of bread. It can be cooked alongside Lamb Casserole (see page 121) to serve at a mixed feast. A lighter stew in summer could contain courgettes, peas and runner beans.

- *1kg (2¼lb) mix of onion, carrot, potato, swede, parsnip, sprouts, beetroot, celery, butternut squash, mushroom, cauliflower, cabbage, peeled and roughly chopped*
- *oil, for frying*
- *2 garlic cloves (optional)*
- *1 tbsp tamari or soy sauce*
- *1 tbsp tomato purée*
- *2 tbsp finely chopped herbs – rosemary, thyme, sage*
- *vegetable stock or water*
- *salt and pepper*

Lightly fry the vegetables together for 5 minutes. Add the garlic (if using), tamari or soy sauce and tomato purée and fry for 3 more minutes, turning frequently. Add the herbs and seasoning. Just cover with stock or water.

Clap on a lid and simmer for 30 minutes or so until vegetables are just done. Rest the stew before serving.

Any leftovers can be blended to make a thick soup.

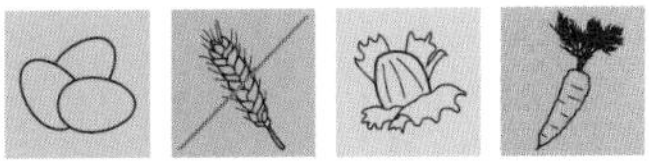

Cake for celebrations

oven

serves 4–8

Everyone needs to celebrate and this is the perfect cake for most people. For vegan friends serve Bonvive Balls (see page 39) or Vegan Cheesecake (see page 33) and enjoy yourselves.

This mix without the nuts is good as a topping on fruit such as blackberries and apples to make a cobbler-type pudding.

- *175g (6oz) spelt or gluten-free flour*
- *2 tsp baking powder*
- *½ tsp bicarbonate of soda (baking soda)*
- *1 tsp ground spice – nutmeg or cinnamon*
- *½ tsp salt*
- *50g (2oz) chopped walnuts (optional)*
- *110g (4oz) sultanas (optional)*
- *1 tsp vanilla paste or 1 finely chopped vanilla pod*
- *125g (4½oz) fat (e.g., coconut oil)*
- *125g (4½oz) sugar or coconut sugar*
- *2 large eggs*
- *4 small ripe bananas*

Heat the oven to 180°C/ fan160°C/350°F/Gas 4. Grease and line a cake tin.

In a large bowl, combine the flour, baking powder, soda, spice and salt. Stir in the walnuts and sultanas , if using, and vanilla.

Beat the fat, sugar and eggs together in a bowl and mash the bananas into them. Add to the flour mix and beat until all is well combined. Pour into the tin and bake for around 1¼ hours until golden and a skewer inserted in the middle of the cake comes out clean.

A UK study involving over 1,500 children has suggested that 10 per cent of children aged between 8 and 16, now identify as vegetarian or vegan, while 44 per cent are trying to eat less meat.

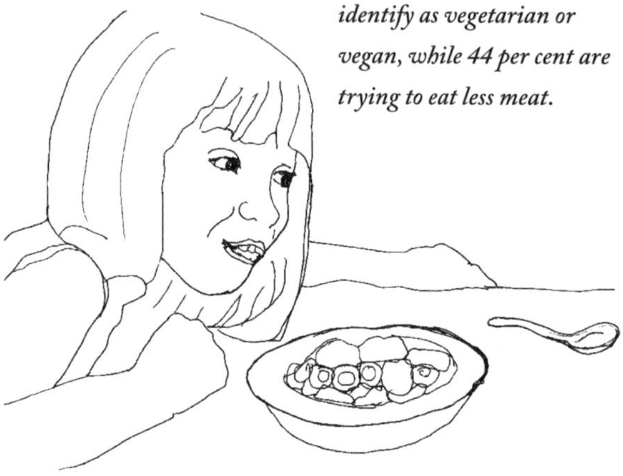

VEGANS

Vegans have chosen their way of eating for many reasons and, if you are a meat eater, it is important for you to realise that people who are vegan are not vegan just to piss you off!

Sometimes people are vegan because they were raised that way and it feels natural and they feel fine. Some people are on a recovery diet, and some just do not like meat.

Other people become vegan for political or moral reasons, which you don't have to agree with or try to argue them out of.

When feasting with people who are vegan, all you have to do is keep the spoons and pans separate and make them a meal without meat or animal products. So, no honey, gelatine, eggs, milk, butter, cheese, dairy spread; no beef, lamb, pork, chicken or other meats; no fish or shellfish. It also means no fish sauce or Oxo stock cubes.

Recently I have seen Facebook memes which picture vegans as aggressive bullies or as weak souls who need a good feed. You would find both these extremes in any population, whatever the diet, so undoubtedly some of them fit the bill. But for the most part vegans are as normal as anyone else and, probably, a bit smarter than me.

Also, people who are vegan are used to being flexible, so an onion and carrot stew will do them if nothing else is available, as long as it has been well flavoured with herbs and Vegemite or miso.

Oh, and the pleasure they show when they realise you have thought about them is very rewarding to see.

Helen

As a young teenager Helen decided she would be vegan after helping a friend sort out her animal rights' magazines. The pictures of poor animals suffering vivisection had quite destroyed her appetite for meat.

We visited my parents and my mum had cooked steak for the family and, as a concession to Helen, a small chicken dish.

'What do you mean it's meat? Well, would you like some fish instead?' she demanded.

Helen burst into tears and fled the table.

My mum learned to cook by cooking meat and two veg, and for her meat meant red meat: lamb, beef and pork, but not chicken and not fish, which was food for invalids. After a bit of explaining and exclaiming how good the food was, my mum calmed down and Helen was coaxed back to the party with a plate of chips and two veg.

It takes patience on both sides to explain this still relatively new phenomenon of veganism to older people.

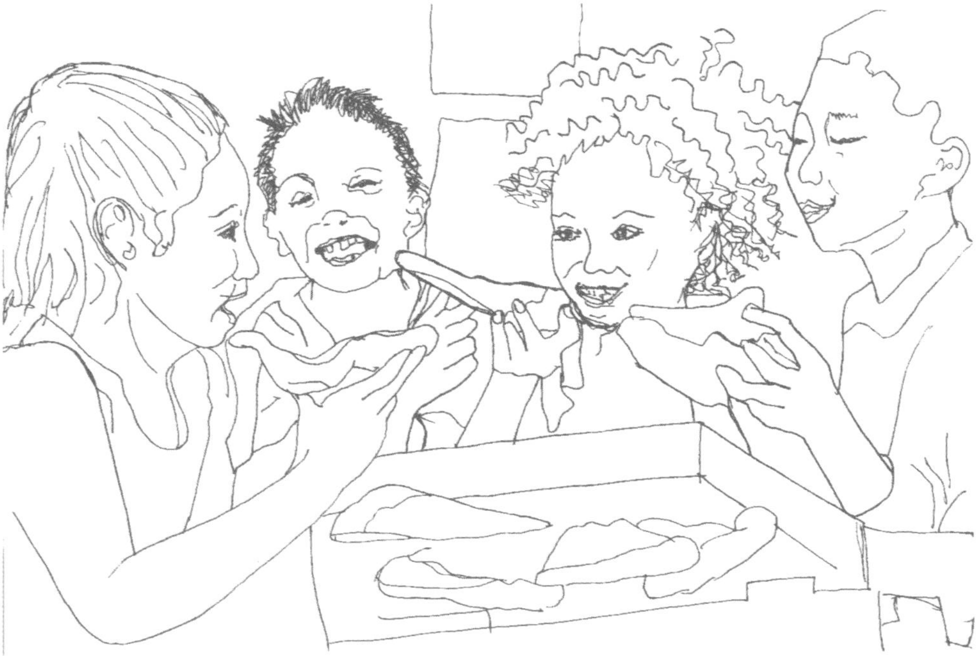

I got this from the Vegan Dalai Lama Pizza Palace. I told them to make me one with everything!

New Zealand potluck

To celebrate the turn of the year, friends of ours in New Zealand had what is called a potluck. Potluck is a gathering where everyone brings one savoury dish and one sweet.

This time, with so many people who could be vegan or vegetarian, it was decided to make everything vegan-friendly.

This turned out to be a huge challenge for many. Emails and phone calls flurried between guests as they decided what could or could not be brought to the table. The meal was a great success and everyone agreed that vegan cooking was quite tasty after all and not too hard, once you got your head around the ingredients.

Norah's tomato soup was particularly savoury, but she warned everyone that she had used a stock cube to give it a little more 'beef'. The vegetarians and vegans all avoided it. Later she confessed, 'Oh, and I added just a little bacon too, but not so much that you would notice it.'

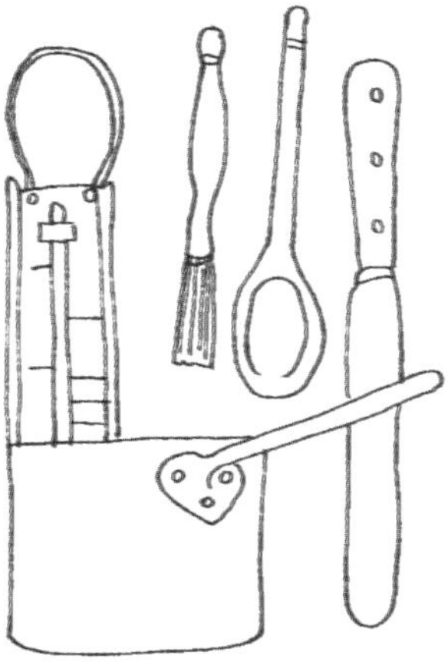

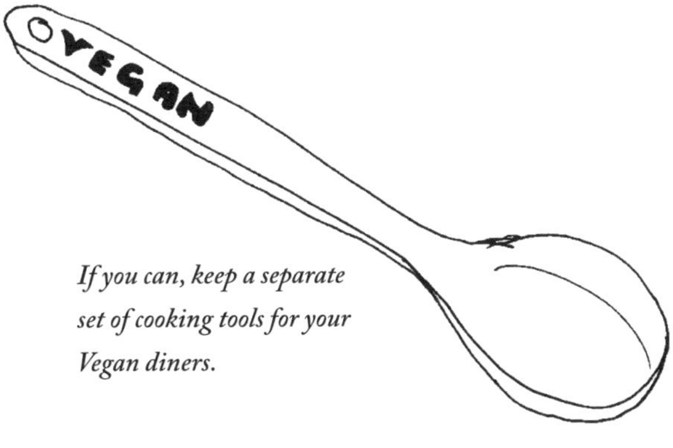

If you can, keep a separate set of cooking tools for your Vegan diners.

RECIPES

Egg substitute – Aquafaba

This is a good egg substitute, but not recommended for those with IBS or IBD.

The juice from a tin of chickpeas can be used as substitute for egg when binding savoury dishes – 3 tablespoons are equivalent to one large egg.

There are many recipes online that use aquafaba. It can even be used to make meringues.

Tahini sauce

serves 4

A tasty, easy sauce for falafels or chickpea patties.

- *4 tbsp tahini*
- *4 tbsp water*
- *1 tsp lemon juice (optional)*
- *salt and pepper*

In a jar, mix the tahini and the water and add some seasoning and the lemon juice. Stir, then shake, until all combined. Add more water to thin if needed.

Falafels

stove top

serves 4

Falafels make a wonderful change from veggie burgers especially in a pitta bread with tahini sauce and chilli relish.

- *1 x 400g tin of chickpeas*
- *1 red onion, finely chopped*
- *1 garlic clove, pressed*
- *1 tsp finely chopped parsley*
- *1 tsp ground cumin*
- *1 tsp ground coriander*
- *1 tsp harissa (optional)*
- *2 tbsp gram flour, plus 4 tbsp for dusting*
- *oil, to shallow fry*

Drain and dry the chickpeas, reserving the aquafaba for another dish.

Mash all the ingredients in a mouli or blend them all together. Press the mix together and add more gram flour if needed to form a stiff dough.

On a plate, with your floured hands, mould the mix into 4cm (1½in) discs, using more gram flour to further firm and coat them.

Fry one in the oil in a pan to check if it will hold together. If it doesn't, add more gram flour, press firmly and try again. Shallow fry the discs in batches until golden brown on all sides.

Drain and store on a sheet of kitchen towel until all are done.

Serve on flatbreads with tahini sauce (see left) and salad.

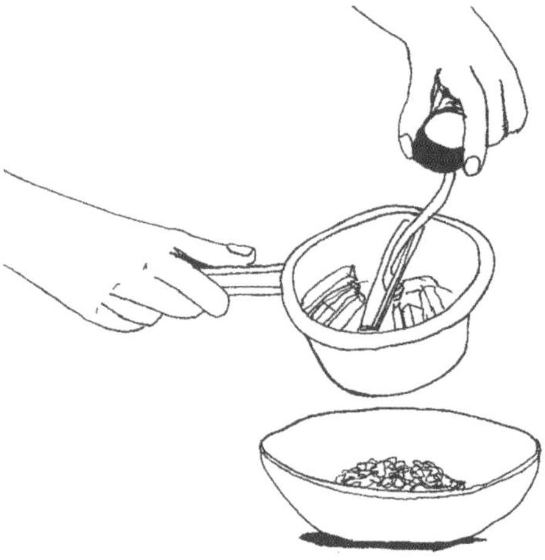

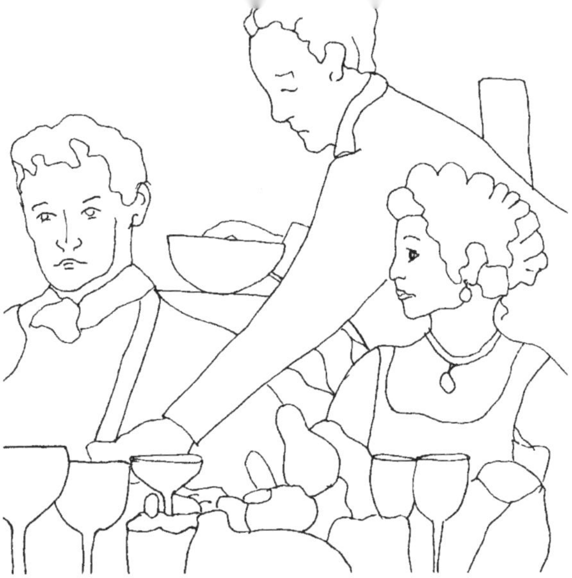

How rare would you
like your steak?

Oh, endangered please

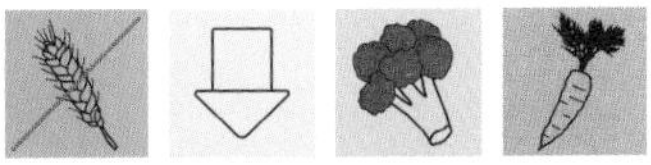

Hummus version 2

serves 4

This white bean version adds a bit of variation to the usual hummus recipe. This hummus can be used to accompany braised tofu and salad.

- *1 x 400g tin of cooked white beans, drained and twice rinsed*
- *2 garlic cloves*
- *2 tbsp tomato purée*
- *1 tsp smoked paprika (optional)*
- *1 tsp cider vinegar*
- *1 tbsp olive oil*
- *1 tsp finely chopped parsley*
- *salt and pepper*

Blend all the ingredients until smooth. Add a little more vinegar or water if it looks too thick. Set to one side to mature for an hour or so and dress with parsley before serving.

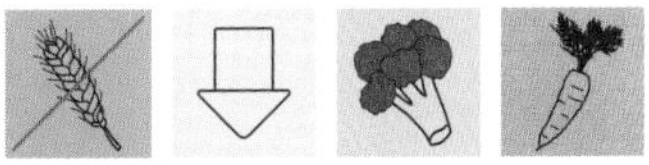

Ribboned leeks

stove top

serves 4

A little gift of a dish which looks beautiful as a special meal accompaniment or perfect for a special lunch.

- *450g (1lb) baby leeks*
- *pinch of salt*
- *melted butter or olive oil, for brushing*

Separate out the white part of the leeks and cut into 6cm (2½in) strips. Divide them into even bundles and wrap each with a strip of the green.

Steam for 4–5 minutes until just soft, then season. Brush with butter or oil and serve on a dish.

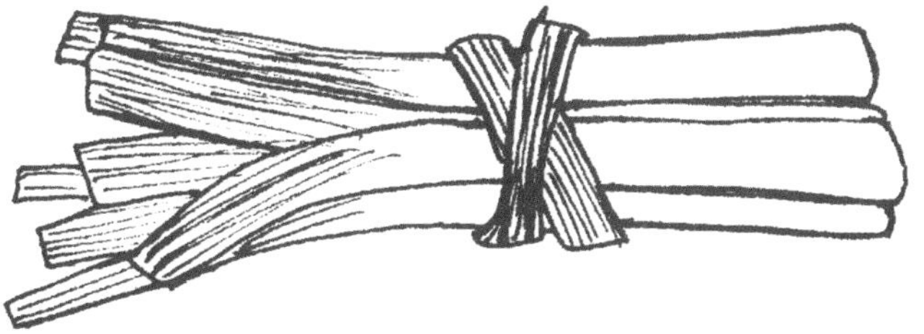

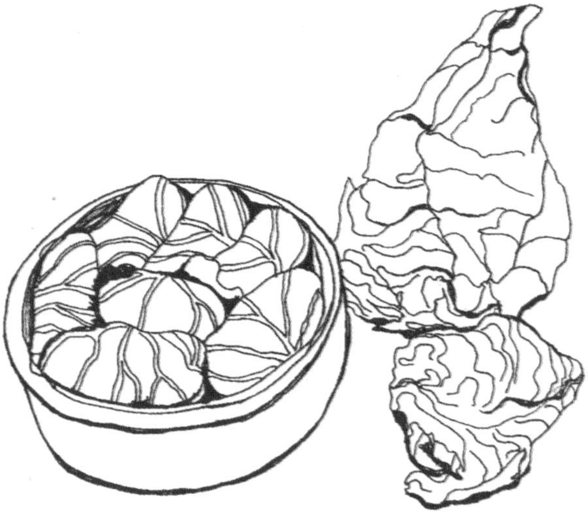

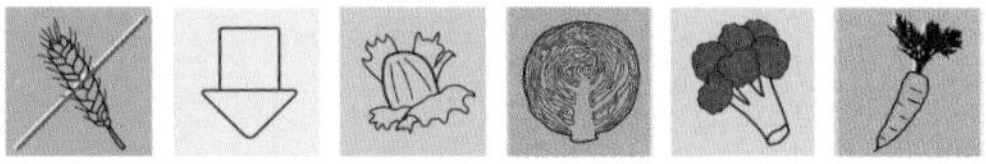

Nut pâté

serves 4–6

This is a great spread for vegans and non-vegans alike. Made in minutes and eaten over several days, it gets tastier as it matures.

- *100g (3½oz) sunflower seeds*
- *100g (3½oz) pumpkin seeds*
- *100g (3½oz) hazelnuts, almonds or cashew nuts (optional)*
- *3 tbsp tomato purée*
- *3 tbsp olive oil*
- *3 garlic cloves, minced*
- *1 tbsp mild curry powder*
- *1 tbsp ground turmeric*
- *salt and pepper*

Blend all the nuts and seeds in a blender until fine.

In a bowl, with a large spoon, combine with all the other ingredients and season to taste. If it seems dry add a little more oil.

Press the mix into a serving bowl and refrigerate (if possible, overnight) before using.

Serve on crackers or toast.

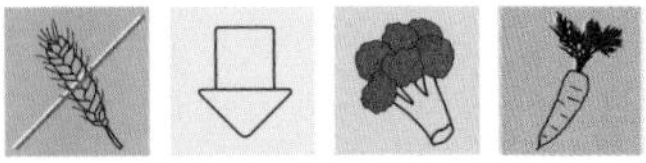

Dolmades with cabbage leaves

stove top & oven

per person

These can be made with leftover rice. Meat-eaters can use cooked and seasoned minced lamb instead of rice. If you are cooking for both vegans and meat-eaters make the vegan dolmades first and keep them separate.

- *3–4 small cabbage leaves*
- *1 tbsp cooked rice per cabbage leaf*
- *1 tbsp chopped mint or basil*
- *finely chopped preserved lemon or 1 tsp lemon juice (optional)*
- *salt and pepper*

Clean the cabbage leaves and cut off any large stalk. Simmer the cabbage leaves for 5 minutes until they soften, then cool.

In a bowl, mix the remaining ingredients together for the filling and season to taste.

Take a leaf and place about 1 tablespoon of rice at one edge. Fold the sides in and roll the leaf until it is a little parcel.

Steam all the parcels together for 10 minutes and serve hot or cold. Or you can lay the dolmades in an oiled baking dish and cover with tomato or Nomato sauce (see page 30) and bake for 30 minutes in an oven at 180°C/fan160°C/350°F/Gas 4. Serve hot.

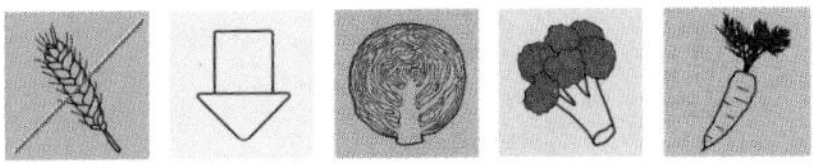

Pesto

serves 4–6

Fresh pesto, like fresh pasta, is a wonderful thing. Combine the two and it tastes heavenly. This pesto will lift any ordinary pasta dish. Add to pizzas or sauces or serve on pasta.

- *150g (5oz) of any chopped leafy herbs – ransoms (spring garlic), basil, sorrel, rocket (arugula)*
- *1– 2 chopped garlic cloves*
- *salt and pepper*
- *1 tbsp lemon juice (optional)*
- *1 tbsp maple syrup (optional)*
- *150ml (5fl oz) olive oil*

Blend all the ingredients together to a smooth paste. Add a little water or oil if it is very dry. Use immediately, or you can freeze this in small batches in an ice-cube tray and bag up.

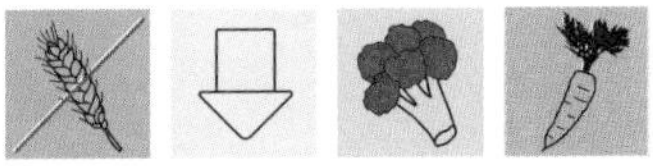

Buckwheat wraps

stove top

serves 4

Not just gluten free, these wraps are particularly nutritious and tasty. Buckwheat provides a good source of protein for vegan diets.

Makes 4 x 20cm (8in) wraps

- *100g (3½oz) buckwheat flour*
- *1 egg or flax egg*
- *100ml (3½fl oz) tepid water*
- *1 tbsp olive or rapeseed oil, plus extra for frying*
- *salt and pepper*

In a bowl combine all the ingredients (except the frying oil) and whisk to a smooth batter. Add a little more water if the batter is very thick.

Brush a heavy frying pan with oil and drop a large spoonful of batter in the centre.

Scrape gently and tip the pan to make a thin round of batter in the base of the pan. It will not run by itself. Fry for 3 minutes either side.

Remove from the pan and stack the wraps in a clean tea towel until serving.

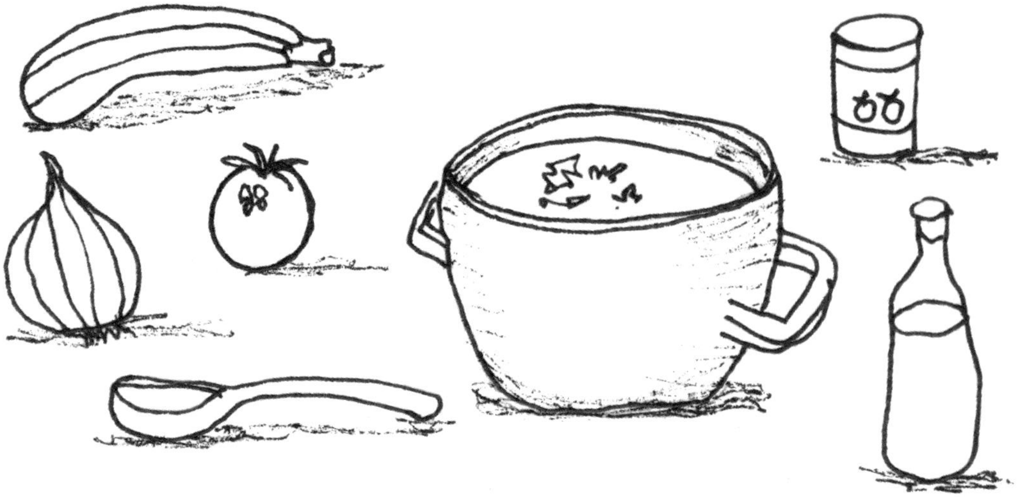

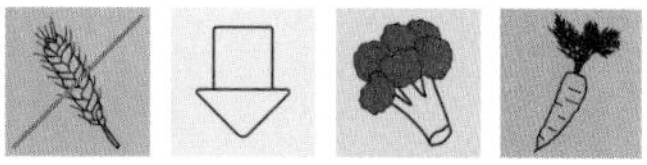

Norah's soup

stove top

serves 4–6

A delicious soup to share at a gathering or as a quick evening meal. This also makes a quick tomato sauce for pasta by using less water and adding a spoonful of pesto.

- *2 onions, grated*
- *2 courgettes (zucchini), grated*
- *1 tbsp oil*
- *¼ tube tomato purée*
- *1 tsp tamari or soy sauce*
- *1 x 400g tin of tomatoes*
- *1 tsp dried mixed herbs*
- *500ml (18fl oz) stock or water and 1 tsp bouillon*
- *salt and pepper*

Sauté the onions and courgettes in the oil for 5–8 minutes. Stir in the tomato purée and tamari or soy sauce and fry for 5 minutes. Add the tinned tomatoes and herbs and stir in the stock or water and bouillon and simmer for 10 minutes.

Leave to cool and blend to a smooth soup. Adjust the seasoning and serve hot.

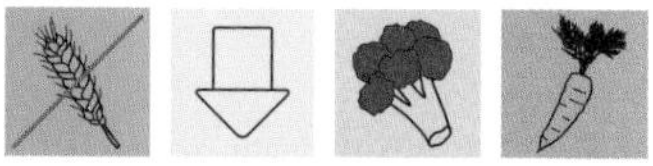

Vegetable soup

stove top

serves 4–6

Vegetable soup doesn't have to be boring. This is a versatile recipe where you can add other ingredients. Try adding whole tomatoes, chunks of braised tofu or fried mushrooms or make dumplings to float on top. As an alternative, add 3 tablespoons of rinsed red lentils, 100ml (3½fl oz) more water and 1 teaspoon of cumin powder.

- *1 carrot, diced*
- *2 onions, chopped*
- *2 celery sticks, chopped*
- *½ swede, diced*
- *2 garlic cloves, minced*
- *1 tbsp chopped rosemary, thyme and sage*
- *1 tbsp tamari or soy sauce*
- *1 tbsp oil for frying*
- *enough stock or water to cover*
- *salt and pepper*

Sauté the carrot, onions, celery and swede together. Add the rest of the ingredients and cover with stock or water and season. Add more liquid for a thinner soup.

When all the vegetables are soft, either mash with a potato masher or blend for a thick, smooth soup.

Serve with warm bread.

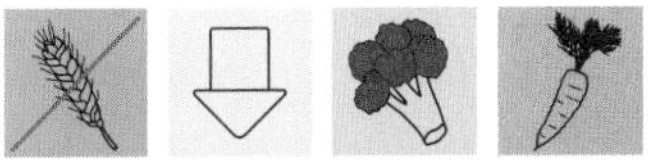

Burger 2 – red lentils & buckwheat

stove top

serves 4

BBQs or fry ups often mean people who are vegan have to eat boring veggie burger. This is a better burger and you can add different spices and herbs to make your own more exotic version.

- *110g (4oz) dried red lentils*
- *110g (4oz) buckwheat seeds*
- *1 tsp dried basil*
- *1 tsp tamari*
- *110g (4oz) gram flour*
- *oil, for frying*
- *sauces (ketchup or mayo type)*
- *burger buns or large lettuce leaves*
- *salt and pepper*

Simmer the lentils for 20 minutes until mushy. At the same time, simmer the buckwheat seeds for about 10 minutes until just mushy.

Drain well and mash the lentils and buckwheat together with basil and some seasoning.

Add about half the gram flour to thicken the mix until stiff. Add more if needed to make it firm enough. Coat your hands with gram flour and shape the mix into burgers. Fry on both sides until crispy and golden.

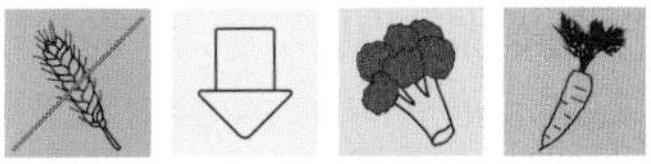

Burger 3 – spiced potato mash

stove top

serves 4

Another take on the burger and this one is packed with flavour. This mash can also be used as a side dish or as a pasty filling.

- *1 tsp cumin seeds*
- *1 tsp mustard seeds*
- *1 tbsp oil*
- *4 potatoes, finely chopped*
- *1 carrot, finely chopped*
- *1 small onion, finely diced*
- *2 tsp curry powder*
- *burger buns*
- *salt and pepper*

Heat the cumin and mustard seeds in a frying pan, then add the oil and all the other ingredients.

On a low heat, fry until the potatoes are crispy on the outside. Mix occasionally to prevent burning.

Add the curry powder. Cool and mash in the pan. Form into burger shapes on a greaseproof paper-lined baking tray. Sometimes the burger falls apart, so be sure to press it together well.

Grill for 5 minutes and serve hot on a bun with sauce of choice.

TOP TIPS

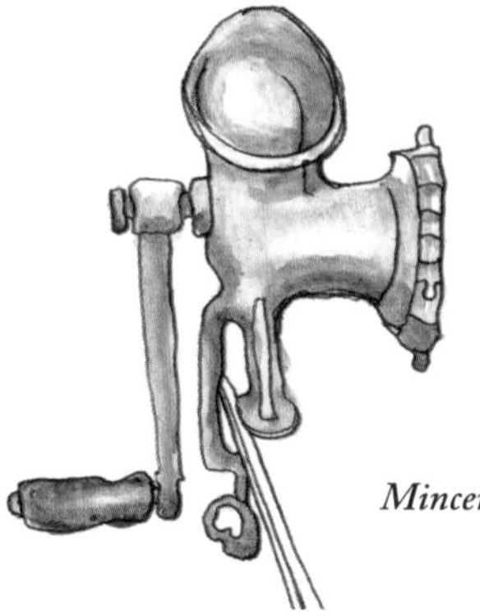

Mincer

Buying local and seasonal if you don't garden

- Ask friends where they get their veg
- Ask friends if they have produce to spare, sell or swap for time in the garden
- Get a veg box
- Look online for local markets
- Buy from roadside home stands
- Buy vegetables that are in season and freeze them, either from fresh or cooked

For the kitchen

- Buy a hand spiralizer
- Buy a mincer
- Buy an efficient blender
- Save plastic ketchup bottles to re-use for pancake batter, salad dressings, drizzles and mayonnaises
- Keep separate implements and a couple of pans, plates and bowls for people with allergies, or who are vegan. Ask them to bring their own eating things
- Use beeswax cloth with specific patterns to wrap and store ingredients for gastro divergent people

Organic gardening

- Buy organic seeds
- Join Garden Organic
- Become a seed saver. Join the Heritage Seed Collection

Join a local gardening club or go to local events

- Look out for a Seedy Sunday, near you
- Buy plants and seedlings from local markets
- Herbs do well on a light window sill. Remember to water them!

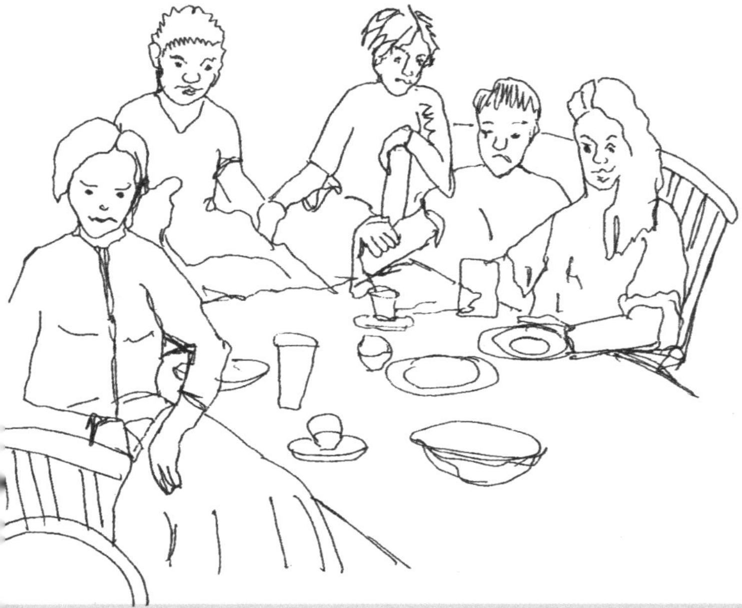

Meat

- Look online for organic meat deliveries or talk to your local butchers or farmers
- Buy from the farmers market

Fish

- Buy local fish in season and freeze; e.g. mackerel will freeze well if airtight

Eat local, feed your community

- Use what you have in the fridge and the cupboard before buying special ingredients.
- Substitute ingredients if you can; e.g. sweet potato for squash and vice versa
- Buy locally and eat out locally at places that use local produce

Be creative

- Read the recipe all the way through
- Decide if you need more information and look online for variations
- If you can, combine some steps or substitute ingredients
- Invent your own recipes on the spot
- Challenge your recipe knowledge. Add a new one a month and cook it three or four times until you know it. Then add some different ingredients or seasoning
- Make recipes and foods a dinner-time conversation. Share with friends and family

INDEX

Acknowledgements

Firstly, my apologies to all the people I unintentionally leave out of this list.

This book started with its title, and I want to thank everyone who said: That's a good title, what's the book about? thus nudging me into writing.

I would like to thank Andy Freedman for encouraging me to tell him about my idea for a book. Then he told the publisher about it! Which brings me to Martin Large of Hawthorn Press, who has my thanks for keeping my name on file.

Katy Bevan, commissioning editor at Hawthorn, found my name and my idea and led me along the path of publication, helping me whenever I needed her. A huge thanks to you Katy.

I'd like to thank Helena Caldon, the recipe editor, who made sense of my erratic weights and measures, oven temperatures and timings.

Thanks too, to the designer, Chris Bailey who turned my raw ideas into a fully baked book and made it so much better than I imagined it would be.

My family always has my love, but many thanks also go to Rod for tea and support. Diolch yn fawr i Josie, Meg, Wil and Bethan, and the in-laws and grandchildren for love and laughs, and for your recipes and for letting me tell your stories.

Gratitude to friends in my wider community for sharing the testing of the recipes and thanks to all who shared tales of their digestive health.